T0095317

fP

Also by Dr. Jennifer Trachtenberg

Good Kids, Bad Habits:
The RealAge Guide to Raising Healthy Children

Also by The Joint Commission and Joint Commission
Resources, with Mehmet C. Oz and Michael F. Roizen

YOU: The Smart Patient: An Insider's Handbook
for Getting the Best Treatmet

The Smart Parent's Guide to Getting Your Kids Through Checkups, Illnesses, and Accidents

EXPERT ANSWERS TO THE QUESTIONS PARENTS ASK MOST

Jennifer Trachtenberg, MD,
with Ron Geraci and Eileen Norris

Also with The Joint Commission,
Joint Commission Resources, and RealAge

Free Press
NEW YORK   LONDON   TORONTO   SYDNEY

Free Press
A Division of Simon & Schuster, Inc.
1230 Avenue of the Americas
New York, NY 10020

Copyright © 2010 by Joint Commission Resources,
RealAge, and Jennifer Trachtenberg, MD

All rights reserved, including the right to reproduce this book or portions
thereof in any form whatsoever. For information address Free Press Subsidiary
Rights Department, 1230 Avenue of the Americas, New York, NY 10020

First Free Press trade paperback edition March 2010

FREE PRESS and colophon are trademarks of Simon & Schuster, Inc.

For information about special discounts for bulk purchases,
please contact Simon & Schuster Special Sales at
1-866-506-1949 or business@simonandschuster.com.

The Simon & Schuster Speakers Bureau can bring authors to your live event.
For more information or to book an event contact the Simon & Schuster Speakers
Bureau at 1-866-248-3049 or visit our website at www.simonspeakers.com.

Manufactured in the United States of America

10   9   8   7   6   5   4   3   2   1

Library of Congress Cataloging-in-Publication Data

Trachtenberg, Jennifer.
    The smart parent's guide to getting your kids through checkups, illnesses,
and accidents : expert answers to the questions parents ask most /
by Jennifer Trachtenberg with Ron Geraci and Eileen Norris.
        p.   cm.
    1. Children—Health and hygiene—Popular works.   I. Geraci, Ron, 1970–
II. Norris, Eileen.   III. Title.
RJ61.T725   2010
618.92—dc22   200905354

ISBN 978-1-4391-5291-1
ISBN 978-1-4391-7189-9 (ebook)

Note to Readers

This publication contains the opinions and ideas of its authors. This publication is intended to provide helpful and informative material on the subjects addressed in the publication. It is sold with the understanding that the authors and publisher are not engaged in rendering medical, health, or any other kind of personal professional services in the book. The reader should consult his or her medical, health, or other competent professional before adopting any of the suggestions in this book or drawing inferences from it.

Please note that this book addresses some topics that The Joint Commission has not studied and about which it has no official positions. For example, The Joint Commission is not an expert on pediatric medicine.

In certain instances, this book lists websites and products by their brand names (such as websites you can go to for help and updated information, and medications), because the authors believe that is how this information will be most helpful to you. The authors have also included names of companies and products on occasion, if they thought that mentioning the name provided relevant information to you. To their knowledge, the authors have no connection to any of the companies, websites, or brand-name products listed in the book, with the exception of RealAge, Inc., the company for which Jennifer Trachtenberg, MD, serves as chief pediatric officer (www.RealAge.com). The authors of the Foreword, RealAge cofounder Dr. Michael Roizen and Dr. Mehmet Oz, also serve on the RealAge Scientific Advisory Board. Furthermore, the inclusion in this book of any specific commercial products or services provided by any specific individual or company in no way constitutes an endorsement by the authors, the publisher, or their affiliates.

The authors and publisher specifically disclaim all responsibility for any liability, loss or risk, personal or otherwise, that is incurred as a consequence, directly or indirectly, of the use and application of any of the contents of this book.

For Max and his smart parents

Contents

Foreword

Michael F. Roizen, MD, and Mehmet C. Oz, MD

This book comes to you from a dynamic duo. No, not Batman and Robin. We're talking about Dr. Jennifer Trachtenberg and The Joint Commission. Dr. Jen is one crazy good pediatrician who is great at helping parents rear healthy kids, but more about her in a moment.

The other half of this team is not a household name, but you should know about The Joint Commission, preferably before your child knocks his head silly and you need to get to the emergency room in the middle of the night. It's critical to go to the *right* hospital, and that's where The Joint Commission comes into the equation. It is the gatekeeper to safety in hospitals and other health care organizations around the world. The Joint Commission evaluates the care, treatment, and services provided to patients and then *accredits* those organizations that meet its very rigorous standards. Let's just say that when you see its seal of approval on a hospital, it means the place and the people who work there have earned your confidence. That's important to you because it means the hospital is going all out to give solid and safe care. This organization really has chops, so trust us when we tell you it's a group that has earned your respect and thanks. That's why we hooked up with The Joint Commission to write *YOU: The Smart Patient* just a few years ago. Like us, The Joint Commission is looking out for you.

Reading about staying healthy can be entertaining. In fact, it's our personal opinion that health books *should* be fun. Dr. Jen and The Joint Commission do a great job of showing you how to make smart choices about your child's health care without turning the pages into a comic book experience. This *Smart Parent's Guide* will help you figure out, for instance, how to find the right pediatrician for your child. It will make you more comfortable about coping with conditions or, God forbid, disease. It will even give you some pointers on how to keep the TV off and make sure the "fast food" your kids eat is dominated by fruit and veggie slices rather than French fries and chicken wings. Then there's the really serious info, like how to get through a hospital visit without having your kid pick up someone else's germs at the hospital or losing your mind (or their life).

When we were looking for a star pediatrician to be the child expert for RealAge.com, we sought Dr. Jen. That was more than six years ago, and it was one of the best connections we have ever made. We trust her in all matters kidlike, and you should too.

We think you'll like the way she and The Joint Commission approach the topic of kids' health care. Besides seeing a bazillion kids every week as a pediatrician and being a mom to three kids, Dr. Jen is also chief pediatric officer for RealAge.com and the respected author of *Good Kids, Bad Habits*. As the brain trust behind the RealAge.com Parenting Center, she helps parents raise healthy kids through the RealAge Healthy Kids Test. (You'll read more about that inside.) She's our go-to pediatrician for anything that has to do with kids. We not only like her expertise, we really like the way she doctors. She's smart (that word again), caring, and friendly, and that comes across whether you see her in her office with patients or making the rounds on the national morning talk shows.

She keeps it real, and you can relate to her just like her patients and their parents do. She gets it, and makes sure her patients and their parents do too. She is the Dr. Mom to many.

Some even say she's the modern-day Dr. Spock, but with a dose of your best gal pal next door. In a nutshell, she will help you grow healthy kids.

Dr. Jen and The Joint Commission are by your side for that amazing parenting roller coaster that is so absolutely wonderful and frustrating and scary and exhilarating. Buckle up and enjoy the ride. And thanks for choosing to be smart about your kids' health.

Introduction

As a pediatrician, I am the best buddy and confidante for the parents of my patients. Want to know one of the most common confessions I hear from parents? They're scared. Sometimes terrified. From caring for a teeny-tiny newborn to coping with a child's medical crisis, they're afraid they'll make a horrible mistake. Good parents like you want to do everything right for their kids.

But a little bit of fear is a good thing. It keeps you on your toes—it makes you question, focus, and think. When it comes to your kids' health, being blissfully unaware can have devastating consequences. As a pediatrician and a mom of three, I've seen the good, the bad, and the very ugly on both sides of the stethoscope. I know the goofs that even ultra-intelligent parents can make and the mistakes that happen in even the best hospitals. Modern medicine can work wonders, but it can also do real harm, thanks to human errors and mechanical breakdowns.

That said, the last thing I want is to paralyze you with fear and worry. A much smarter strategy—one that I use myself and encourage you to use as well—is to *use* fear to your advantage. Treat being scared as a signal that you need to know more. The

 1 in 15 children in hospitals is injured by medical mistakes and adverse drug reactions.

more you know, the smarter the decisions you'll make about your children's health. Yes, you're right, *there's so much information out there that a person could drown in it.* So what's the best way to navigate this vast sea of new medical knowledge you're blessed (and burdened) with?

That's why I wrote this book: to give you my insider's recommendations on how to **protect your child's health.** Because that's your most important mission as a parent.

Don't feel compelled to read this book straight through. You're a parent. You don't have much extra time on your hands, do you? Take a spin through chapter 1 whenever you need to give your child a medication, even a simple fever reducer. Read chapters 2 and 3 so you know how to find the right pediatrician and how to keep your kids healthy. And read chapter 4 so that you're prepared for the unexpected. Otherwise, open it when you start to feel that uneasy sense of fear creeping in but before you're in a full-blown panic.

When it is your child's turn to go to the hospital, you shouldn't leave *anything* to chance. As a doctor, I've seen too many things go wrong from the start. You need to be more vigilant about your child's care in the hospital than anywhere. And you'll likely have to be at your best when you're nearly at your wit's end and would rather become a dumbfounded bystander.

It happens to thousands of parents every day.

But don't let it happen to you.

I want to give you tips on how to hold it together and make things go right, because I have truly been there and done that. This book provides the inside strategies that I use to get good results and avoid critical, common blunders where it matters

 If you live in the U.S., the odds that your child will be hospitalized this year are **1 in 25.**

most—in the emergency department, pediatrics ward, all-night pharmacy, exam room, or any other medical hot spot where your child's health can be on the line. While there are plenty of books loaded with children's health advice—believe me, I own them all—none approaches health care quite like this field guide does. It will help you make the *right* decisions, whether you're just trying to get the best care for your child during a routine office visit or you're in the middle of a full-blown health crisis.

The great team behind this book will also help you. My co-authors include The Joint Commission—a not-for-profit organization that accredits and certifies more than seventeen thousand hospitals, health care organizations, and programs in the United States—and RealAge, a health company that provides some of the most useful free tests on the Internet, including its Healthy Kids Test. (I'm its chief pediatric officer.) Collaborating with these two organizations has yielded insights that you'll find in no other book.

The experts at The Joint Commission impart wisdom that you'll find invaluable (as I have) in choosing the best hospital for your child. (That's a mission you should start *right now,* by the way; see page 166 to learn why.) The Joint Commission evaluates hospitals and other health care organizations to ensure that they meet top-quality standards in care, cleanliness, and procedures—and when hospitals fall short, it works to get them fixed. The Joint Commission strives to fulfill its vision that "all people always experience the safest, highest quality, best-value health care across all settings."

You may know The Joint Commission by way of *YOU: The Smart Patient,* the bestseller that it produced with two lovable guys whom I'll bet you're familiar with: Michael Roizen, MD, and Mehmet Oz, MD. Known to millions as the "YOU Docs," these physician-authors have changed countless lives through their books, TV appearances, and radio programs. They also wrote the foreword to this book. Thanks, guys!

As a parent, you work hard to teach your kids not to do certain risky things, from running with scissors to sending their e-mail address to a stranger. Moms and dads need expert guidelines too, especially when it comes to their kids' health. This book will give you my rules for dealing with the medical system—the kinds of tips that could save your child's life one day. Even tomorrow.

And remember, it's okay to be a little scared. It's the sure sign of a smart parent.

The Smart Parent's Guide to Getting Your Kids Through Checkups, Illnesses, and Accidents

Chapter 1

When Should You Give Kids Medicine—Or Not?

Making Sure No One—Including You—Gives Your Child the Wrong Thing

POP QUIZ

Do you know how children are medicated? Prove it by acing this quiz—and by acing, I mean answering all six questions correctly without guessing. (Tip: There may be more than one correct answer.) If you get them all right (answers can be found at the end of the chapter), feel free to skip to the next chapter. If not, no worries: You'll find out everything you need to know about safe ways to give kids medications in the pages ahead.

1. When is it okay to give your baby or young child baby aspirin?
   A. For mild headaches, but only for kids four or older
   B. When ibuprofen and acetaminophen have failed to work
   C. Never
   D. When he or she is a baby (duh!)

2. Which of these ailments should be treated with antibiotics?
   A. Colds and flus
   B. Chicken pox (varicella)
   C. German measles (rubella)
   D. None of the above

3. What has been shown to be more effective than many over-the-counter cough suppressants?
   A. M&Ms
   B. Olive oil
   C. Honey
   D. Immersion in an ice-cold bath for three minutes

4. Determining the correct dose of medication for a child is usually based on ...
   A. Weight in kilograms, and some educated guesswork
   B. Weight in pounds, and some educated guesswork
   C. Age, height, and medical history
   D. Blood type

5. What's the disturbing little "secret" that often makes giving a child even a well-known drug somewhat risky?
   A. Almost all the pills prescribed for children don't have an enteric coating, which could cause tongue nodules.
   B. Children's medications are often impure because many are imported from countries with low pharmaceutical-manufacturing standards.
   C. Only a few hundred of the thousands of drugs given to children daily have been clinically tested on kids.

6. What is the best way to dispose of unneeded medications?
   A. Throw them in the garbage.
   B. Flush them down the toilet.
   C. Mix them with coffee grounds or kitty litter, then put the mixture in a sealed bag or empty can, and then put that in the trash.
   D. Take them to the same place where you recycle used printer cartridges.

Most parents are pretty happy when I hand them a prescription for their child. Hey, you didn't drive thirty-five minutes with a crying toddler to go home with a cold compress, right? And if you've ever pulled an all-nighter lying next to a miserable kid waiting for a fever reducer to kick in, you know how to spell relief. Pain relievers can soothe your child's midnight earache and let you *both* get back to sleep . . . children on asthma medicine can breathe easier . . . antiseizure drugs can help control epilepsy . . . and the list goes on. Medications *can* be a beautiful thing.

However, the downsides to medication use in children are many—and they're likelier worse than you think. Every time I write a prescription, I know I'm taking a risk. That's why I double-check every nanodrop, every granule, every *molecule* of medication that I give to my patients and my own children.

Why? Because the tiniest differences—like ingesting 1.5 grams of a drug instead of 1 gram—can be catastrophic in a patient who only weighs eleven pounds. And because when it comes to prescribing drugs for children, pediatricians are still flying semiblind in the majority of cases. It's chiefly an art of "off-label" guesswork. **"Off-label"** is the term used when a doctor prescribes a medication for a purpose or age group that the Food and Drug Administration (FDA) has not approved—in other words, that's not spelled out on the label. Yet off-label prescribing is very common, totally legal, and often excellent medicine.

Scared yet? I'm not trying to make you a paranoid parent, just a smart one. Because misuse of medications—or even a seemingly correct use that exposes children to risks we don't fully understand yet—is a real danger. In rare cases, the consequences can be tragic.

Dirty Little Secrets

When it comes to children and medications, modern science doesn't know much. As unbelievable as it sounds, as many as 75 percent of the drugs docs use on children have never been tested on children. We have good information on only about two hundred of the more common medications. That leaves thousands of both prescription and over-the-counter medications untested in kids. Why? For decades, physicians simply lowered drug dosages for children, on the assumption that humans process drugs identically and kids are just small humans.

Wrong! Children are *not* little adults. Their bodies are not just growing, they are changing and maturing, too. For example, immune systems and nervous systems continue developing through the first several years of a child's life. No wonder kids process drugs differently than adults do and often react to them differently too, even at the lowest dosages.

Yet amazingly, only about half of the new drugs approved every year by the FDA undergo reliable testing in children.

We pay the consequences for this every day. Dosing miscalculations and other errors happen more frequently than any parent would like to imagine, and research shows that 95 percent of the problems go unreported. Still, if you watch the news or surf the Internet, you know that dosing problems in children are common at home and in hospitals, and adverse reactions to drugs are rampant. You've also probably read and heard that many children are overmedicated and many are undermedicated.

All true.

But things are looking up. The U.S. government is working to get pharmaceutical companies to test more medications for children. That's a big change. Historically, the drug companies didn't do trials on kids. It was a matter of both practicality and ethics. Would you volunteer *your* little Bobby to test a new pill so that future children might benefit? If he sprouts a hump on his back as a side effect, would you tell him that you really needed the three hundred bucks you got for volunteering him as a guinea pig?

That's why it's hard to get parental approval for children to participate in studies.

Money is a big driver though. In the past, there wasn't much to be made in pediatric medications compared to adult remedies. Now there are more incentives for the drug companies to study the effects of medications on kids, and so more companies are doing just that.

Why We Go Off-Label

If pediatricians prescribed only drugs approved for kids, we'd have a lot of sick kids. So it's extremely common for doctors to prescribe medications off-label for children. In fact, around 80 percent of medicine used for kids is prescribed off-label.

In some cases, there is good data showing that a particular drug is safe and effective in children, but the pharmaceutical company only applied for FDA approval to use the drug in adults—because each separate approval (adults and kids) is a long, costly process. For example, you probably remember hearing about Prozac being approved for treating kids with depression. Actually, doctors had been prescribing it to children off-label for years. The drug company just had not applied to the FDA for approval for kids until then.

Albuterol, used for asthma, is another good example. Even though it's only approved for kids over two, docs regularly pre-

Mad Scientists?

Some health pundits claim that kids who take a drug that hasn't been studied on children are essentially participating in an "experiment," just without their parents' knowledge. Technically, I suppose that's true. Functionally, it's a necessity, and one that's usually quite safe for your child. Trust me. I prescribe off-label drugs for my own kids when that's the best med.

scribe albuterol for children younger than that if it is needed. *Not* treating asthma is a poor alternative. And albuterol has been used for so long with so much success that it's now generally considered safe.

The downside of a doctor using medications off-label is that pediatricians have to estimate the dosage for kids based on the amount that's been proven effective in adults (or, sometimes, in older children). Pediatricians have a lot of practice at this. But there's always some risk of a child getting too much or too little medicine if the dose isn't calculated correctly, so that's why caution is key: I always give the smallest dose possible to do the job in order to minimize the odds that the drug will cause side effects.

While You're at the Pharmacy, Pick Up a Magnifying Glass

How do you know if your child has been prescribed a medicine off-label? You won't, unless you ask your doctor or pharmacist. Or unless you check the package insert—the printed, teeny, folded piece of paper that comes with the medication—to see what and whom the drug *has* been approved to treat. The FDA is making these descriptions easier to read, but they are still a little academic for the average mom or dad. In the "Indications and Usage" section, you'll see what ages and problems the medication is approved to treat. (Keep in mind we often prescribe medications off-label for conditions not included in the original FDA approval.) Also check out the "Highlights" section at the very end. It will give you a good summary of warnings and precautions, possible adverse reactions, drug interactions, and how to take the medicine (with liquids, without food, etc.). This section is pretty easy to understand.

What Would You Do?

A recent study in a children's hospital found that 77 percent of parents want only FDA-approved treatments for their kids, and only 30 percent would allow their children to take part in clinical studies that involve new treatments. However, if the risk is minimal, 36 percent of all those surveyed would consider participating in clinical trials if their child had the same disease as the one being studied; 25 percent would allow their child to be a healthy volunteer.

The Top Five Medicines I Prescribe for Kids

In a survey of 1,600 pediatricians by the American Academy of Pediatrics, the docs reported they write prescriptions for 53 percent of patients they see in an average week. Among these prescriptions, pediatricians said 73 percent were for "short-term acute illnesses," such as colds and flus, and 29 percent were for "long-term chronic illnesses," such as asthma. In my own practice, here are the top five meds I'm likely to prescribe on any given day:

1. **Amoxicillin.** It's a common antibiotic for ear infections and strep throat, usually given to kids in a bubblegum-pink liquid form. You'll find it in almost every parent's fridge at some point during their children's growing-up years. Fortunately, it tastes pretty good, so kids usually take it without a problem.

2. **Zithromax** (azithromycin). This antibiotic (also known as "Z-Pack") is used for bronchitis and pneumonia; it's also the go-to option for kids who are allergic to penicillin.
3. **Zantac** (ranitidine). This liquid prescription version of the adult heartburn medicine is used for babies with severe spitting-up problems (gastroesophageal reflux).
4. **Albuterol.** It's a bronchodilator, meaning it relieves wheezing or asthma by opening up the airways. I usually prescribe it as an inhaler or in a nebulizer, though liquid forms and tablets are available too.
5. **Ocuflox** (ofloxacin ophthalmic). These are antibiotic drops used to treat pinkeye (conjunctivitis). It seems like every kid gets pinkeye at some point or another and then shares it with their best buddies, and probably with you, too!

When the Best Med Is No Med

If a medication won't help (and often it won't), my job is to explain to parents that a drug isn't necessary—the condition will go away on its own. Sometimes the best medicine for a child is tender loving care, not a prescription, but I'm not always popular when I prescribe TLC rather than a pill. It's not easy to tell a frazzled mom who hasn't slept in twenty hours that what her sick four-year-old needs is coloring books, cartoons, and couch time. But you need to understand that doctors like me are reluctant to prescribe antibiotics when your child's condition won't be helped by them—and when the meds might cause a reaction or complication that's worse than the condition we're trying to treat. (More on this shortly.)

The Catastrophe of Unnecessary Antibiotics

No doubt you've seen the headlines and warnings about overusing antibiotics. They're prescribed unnecessarily to vast numbers of patients every day, typically for viral infections (like colds and flu), on which they have no effect. Let's repeat the chorus: **Antibiotics kill bacteria, not viruses.** When antibiotics are unnecessarily prescribed, it increases the chances bacteria have to "get used to them." The more often bacteria are exposed to commonly used antibiotics, the more likely the bacteria are to mutate and become resistant to these drugs. Mutant bacteria, often termed "superbugs," can be super dangerous because they've learned to shrug off many antibiotics. The statistics are scary: Today, 70 percent of patients who acquire infections in hospitals—where many of these superbugs live—are infected with bacteria that are now resistant to at least one antibiotic that used to kill them.

To the general public, the most alarming consequences of antibiotic abuse are the growing outbreaks of methicillin-resistant *Staphylococcus aureus* (MRSA). In 2005, an estimated 18,650 people died in the U.S. from MRSA. These infections often begin in small scratches or bruises and spread like a forest fire through an infected person's body. Conventional antibiotics are useless to stop them.

If you think MRSA sounds scary, there's a new twist: VRSA. In 2002, the U.S. saw its first case of VRSA, a patient who was infected with a staph strain that was resistant to vancomycin—the powerful, "last-line" antibiotic we typically use only in extreme cases. Since then, a few more cases of VRSA have appeared. Physicians have thrown an arsenal of antibiotics at this superbug, and, luckily, so far it has worked. But unless doctors and patients work together to eliminate all antibiotic abuse, we may soon pine for the good old days when MRSA seemed like our nastiest enemy.

Properly anxious? So am I, as are most physicians. Again, I'm not trying to make you paranoid, just savvy.

The take-home here: Please do *not* twist your doctor's arm to prescribe an antibiotic for your child (or yourself) when it isn't likely to help—and could hurt us all. Here's a general guide to when antibiotics are and aren't warranted.

VIRAL INFECTIONS

Antibiotics are useless against these

Colds and flus

Chicken pox (varicella)

Measles (rubeola)

German measles (rubella)

Roseola infantum (human herpes virus HHV-6 and HHV-7)

"Fifth disease" (parvovirus B19 infection, *Erythema infectiosum*)

Upset stomach/diarrhea (gastroenteritis)

BACTERIAL INFECTIONS

Antibiotics *can* treat these

Most sinus infections

Strep throat

Urinary tract infections

Pneumonia

Most ear infections (otitis media)

Nasty bacterial skin infections (impetigo)

TIP: The FDA offers a website that contains the latest safety information regarding medications. Go to www.fda.gov/cder/drugsafety.htm.

Are We Too Quick to Medicate?

Maybe you've heard the term "Generation Rx," but I'm not sure how apt it really is. In my practice, I don't know of any parents who want their children to be on medication unless they absolutely have to be. At the same time, some lifestyle trends have increased medication use among children. For example, prescriptions for type 2 diabetes drugs in children more than doubled from 2002 to 2005, especially among teen girls. This is largely due to the increase in childhood obesity.

That said, I do know of cases in which children have been put on meds without a sufficient workup to diagnose their condition or to determine if there are alternatives to medication. This is especially true when it comes to psychiatric issues, which can sometimes benefit from talk therapy (though that may take longer). As many as six million children are prescribed psychiatric drugs every year.

There are some children experiencing shyness or stress from peer pressure—which as we all know are just natural parts of growing up—who may be taking psychiatric drugs they don't need, which is a serious issue. However, sometimes a parent's fear of resorting to medication can cause a child to remain undiagnosed and struggle unnecessarily with medical issues. I would never want a child with clinical depression to suffer needlessly if drugs could help. I've also seen kids thrive when put on a medication for ADHD, such as Ritalin (methylphenidate). About 3.5 percent of American children take the drug. Is it wrongly prescribed in some cases? Probably, but there are also many children who aren't taking the drug who would be helped by it. (For more info on ADHD, see page 146.)

My bottom line: Before agreeing to put your child on any long-term drug therapy, make sure a thorough medical evaluation is done (complete medical history, including any behavioral issues) to really get to the root of the problem. It may be a chemical imbalance, and your child may indeed need medications to function well in school and at home. But there may be nondrug alternatives that would also be effective. Investigate all options, and don't hesitate to get a second opinion.

Errors, Mistakes, and Mishaps: When Medications Attack

Medication errors happen for a variety of reasons, but many often come down to one word: math. Yes, your pediatrician (like you) can hit the wrong calculator key, or do the math too fast in his head, or forget to borrow, or run out of fingers. Almost 18 percent of pediatric dosing errors come from math mistakes. Some children are on complex regimens that require a lot of careful calculations based on their weight in kilograms. Their weight determines how many milligrams of the med is needed, then that's converted to how many teaspoons are needed in that particular medicine, which may come in different concentrations. And that's not even figuring in sloppy handwriting! Also, some meds are available only in adult dosages, which must be reformulated or diluted for children. More math.

Finally, kids grow *fast*. A med that was right a few weeks ago may not be now. (I don't know about your kids, but I swear my kids grow inches and add pounds overnight. We've all seen crazy growth spurts.) Plus kids have a varying ability to metabolize medications, and young kids can't always tell you if a medication is actually making them feel sicker. All of these factors can create an accident waiting to happen.

While most pediatric medication mistakes do not result in serious problems, researchers have found that 2.5 percent of them cause significant harm or death. In 2007, the accidental blood thinner overdose of actor Dennis Quaid's newborn twins brought public attention to the issue of pediatric medication errors. In that case, the vials looked the same for infants and adults, but the adult concentration was much higher. Those bottles have since been changed to make it clear which is which. In 2008, The Joint Commission issued an alert aimed at trying to prevent these kinds of mistakes, emphasizing that potentially harmful medication errors occur three times more often in children than in adults. The Joint Commission's alert calls for . . .

- hospitals to weigh children in kilograms when admitted, because weight in kilograms is used to calculate proper doses for children
- doctors to write out how they arrive at a dosage so the math can be double-checked by a pharmacist, nurse, or both
- hospitals to clearly mark medications that have been repackaged from adult doses to kid versions
- hospitals to keep adult meds away from pediatric units and/or to store child and adult medicines in separate areas

Some hospitals are starting to color-code medications by weight ranges for kids, so that if your child weighs between twenty and twenty-four kilograms, for example, his meds might be blue. If doctors needed a lower or higher dose, they would have to make a special request to change that standardized dose. Sounds like a good idea to me.

Preventing Medication Errors in the Doctor's Office

Before you accept any prescription from your pediatrician, I'd ask the following questions:

❏ **"Can you please reweigh my child? I want to be sure what his weight is in kilograms."** As you now know, your child's weight in kilograms is vital because doses are given in milligrams and milliliters. (Oh yes, the jolly metric system, which you have successfully avoided since grade school. Didn't know it was on the smart parent must-know list, did you!) Unfortunately, hurried doctors have been known to wrongly use pounds when calculating doses—and a dose based on 80 pounds instead of 36.3 kilograms will obviously be *way* wrong.

Weight affects how medications are absorbed into the body. It's one reason your pediatrician weighs your child on every office visit. You can also double-check with the pharmacist when picking up a prescription that the dose is appropriate for your child's weight.

❏ **"Rather than one teaspoon, how many *milliliters* are you prescribing?"** No, you won't need to get out your old chemistry set to give your child medicine. Most liquid medicines now come with droppers that display milliliters. Use them! The common assumption that most teaspoons hold around five milliliters of liquid is wrong and dangerous. The average teaspoon varies from two to nine milliliters. So ignore the old Mary Poppins song about a spoonful of sugar helping the medicine go down. Spoons can lead to medication errors. In my experience, by the way, measuring by spoon almost always results in *underdosing,* which prolongs many illnesses.

❏ **"Sorry . . . where precisely is the *decimal point*?"** This insidious math gremlin causes up to half of dosing errors. No kidding. So ask: Is that 1.0 gram or 10 grams? Always clarify the dose with your doctor.

❏ **"Can you show me how you calculated that dosage?"** A classic study a decade ago of sixty-four pediatric residents found that *half* made at least one math error on a ten-question dosing test—and seven made errors that could have caused fatal overdoses. Another reason why you'll see most pediatricians with a calculator in their pocket.

❏ **"Would you read that prescription back to me?"** In one study, up to 25 percent of errors were from confusion caused by medications having similar names. So check and double-check. Er-

> **TIP:** If you're confused about any dose of medicine, prescription or not, ask the doctor or pharmacist to show you how much each dose should be. That's our job—to answer your questions!

rors also happen from poor penmanship (which is why more doctors are turning to computerized prescriptions that are neatly printed out) or because of hard-to-read labels.

❑ **"Do I have to worry about this drug interacting with any foods, other medications, vitamins, or even juice?"** Re-ask the pharmacist, too. See page 26 for more about this.

❑ **"What are you prescribing, in what concentration, how much should my child take, and for how long?"** Make sure your doctor answers this, not just the pharmacist. Pharmacists can make mistakes too. For instance, I had a patient call me and say, "I thought you said to take five milliliters two times a day for ten days? The bottle says ten milliliters twice a day." In this case, the pharmacist didn't tell me or the parent that he filled the prescription with a different concentration because the drugstore was out of what I ordered. Had the patient taken what I originally ordered—one teaspoon—the medicine would not have been effective. Again, always double-check!

> **TIP:** It's actually easy to calculate your child's weight in kilograms. Just take the weight in pounds and divide it by 2.2. For example, if your child weighs 36 pounds, divide 36 by 2.2 to get 16.36 kilograms. (I know it's math—but it's important!)

Be One of the 30 Percent!

A staggering 70 percent of parents dispense medications to their children incorrectly, according to a study from Emory University.

Let's Talk Over-the-Counter Meds

When your child has a cough, a cold, or some other common illness, taking a trip down the drugstore aisle can be overwhelming. The rows and rows of syrups, pills, caplets, elixirs, balms . . . you could waste an hour and get a headache trying to read the labels. Advertising phrases like "clinically proven," "#1 pediatrician recommended," or "all natural" only add to the mental clutter and may not mean much. Worse, you're probably trying to figure this out while you juggle a sick child and a shopping cart.

One of the biggest misconceptions among parents is that over-the-counter meds are safer than prescription meds. They're not. They can be as dangerous. Just one overdose of acetaminophen can be poisonous to the liver, kidneys, and brain, even causing irreversible damage and death—and it's all too easy to give a fussing baby an overdose. Also, docs have known for some time that commonly used cold and cough medications may not be that effective in reducing symptoms in young children and can cause serious complications. Children under two are most vulnerable. Cough and cold meds can cause their hearts to beat too fast and provoke irritability, sleeplessness, and strange behavior—without ever making their noses less runny! I've been telling parents for years about the downside to these medications. They're best avoided. (Find more about cold and cough meds on page 21.)

It's smart to ask your pediatrician and pharmacist for advice

TIP: When your child is taking a medication, jot down the time you give it to him. It's easy to wonder, "Gee, did I give him his pill at ten A.M., or was it eleven? Or, eek, did I forget it?" Writing it down also helps if both Mom and Dad are dispensing meds. Keep a list that either parent completes each time a dose is given.

on over-the-counter medications. A little Q & A can save you hours of regret and cash. When you inspect the labels, you'll find that most products for a similar condition contain the same active ingredients in the same amounts. Don't forget to double-check with your pediatrician and/or pharmacist what the correct dose is based on your child's weight in kilograms. Then make sure you're giving your child exactly that dosage, no more or less.

Ibuprofen or Acetaminophen?

Which pain reliever do you reach for when your child has a fever or an earache or headache? There's a good chance it's the same one your parents gave you. Most contain either ibuprofen (its familiar brand name is Motrin) or acetaminophen (yes, that's Tylenol). While there's no shame in brand loyalty, it may not be the best strategy. Here are my six tips for giving children ibuprofen or acetaminophen.

1. **Never give your child any kind of aspirin (I cannot stress this enough)**—not even baby aspirin, which is *not* for babies. Aspirin can cause Reye's syndrome (see page 31). Many of you might remember taking baby aspirin in your own childhood but that was before anyone knew better. Let me repeat: Baby aspirin is *not* for babies or kids under sixteen.

19

2. **Always treat your child, not the fever.** If your child has a mild fever but appears happy and playful, it is not necessary to give your child a fever reducer. Germs don't like higher body temperatures, so if your child is fighting an infection and does not seem uncomfortable, I'd skip the meds. The immune system has warmed up and is doing its work.

3. **Do not give ibuprofen to infants under six months old or to kids who are dehydrated or vomiting.** It can cause gastritis and stomach pains.

4. **Don't give your child acetaminophen unless you're certain of the dose, and never give it for more than five days in a row.** With care, acetaminophen can usually be given to young kids, even infants, but always check with your pediatrician first. Overdosing can be toxic to the liver, which is one of the most frequent causes of medication-related death in children. Acetaminophen is used to treat mild to moderate pain and fever. It does have the benefit of coming in a suppository form, which can be helpful if your child is vomiting or refusing to take medications by mouth. It doesn't have any anti-inflammatory properties so it's not the best choice for treating muscle aches or sports injuries.

5. **As always, be very careful with dosing.** If you give your child medicine on your own, *always* follow the dosing instructions on the label. In certain situations, your pediatrician might recommend a different dose of ibuprofen or acetaminophen than what the label recommends, depending on your child's condition. In that case, follow your doctor's instructions to the letter.

6. **Don't mix acetaminophen and ibuprofen.** It can be risky to alternate them—especially if a child is dehydrated or has other medical problems—so don't just grab whatever you see first in the medicine cabinet. The drugs can react with each other to cause serious side effects, including kidney damage. If you've already given your child ibuprofen for fever and want to add acetaminophen for pain, check with

FACT: Studies suggest that parents give kids incorrect doses of over-the-counter fever medicine in nearly 50 percent of cases. I know that when your child is miserable or crying, you're trying to help fast, but take an extra minute or two to ensure that the dose is correct.

your pediatrician first. If your doctor okays alternating the two, keep a written schedule so that you give the right one at the right time.

Cough and Cold Meds: An Update

You know those cold medicines the FDA recently nixed for young kids? (It strongly recommended against giving over-the-counter cough and cold products to infants and children under age two.) Apparently, not everyone is heeding that warning. A recent study found that one in ten U.S. children is still being given these meds—even though manufacturers of fourteen major over-the-counter cold and cough products made for babies voluntarily removed their products from the shelves, and despite national media coverage highlighting the risks: serious side effects that include rapid heartbeat, convulsions, loss of consciousness, and even death.

Why are these products so potentially hazardous? In part because many of them contain multiple drugs—a combo of decongestants, for unclogging stuffy noses; expectorants, for loosening mucus; antihistamines, for sneezing and runny noses; and/or antitussives, to quiet coughs. That's four medicines in one dose! That's a lot for a small body to handle.

As of this writing, the FDA has not taken any action since its warning. However, an FDA advisory panel has also recommended against using cold and cough medications for kids aged two to six, while voting not to suggest restrictions for children aged six to twelve. Just so you know, this advisory does not include antihistamines, such as Benadryl (diphenhydramine), for allergies and runny noses. They're okay to take, but talk to your doctor first.

So what should you do for a kid with a miserable cough or cold? I would say (gee, surprise!) talk to your doctor, who will probably recommend the following:

- giving acetaminophen or ibuprofen if your child has a fever
- making sure your child drinks plenty of liquids to avoid dehydration
- using saline nasal drops to loosen mucus (or suction mucus from your child's nose with a bulb syringe)

If you're tempted to do more, keep this statistic in mind: Seven thousand children under age eleven are treated in hospital emergency departments every year for overdoses of nonprescription cough and cold medications. About two-thirds of those cases happened when children took the meds without their parents' knowledge. But in one-quarter of the cases, the parent gave the *correct* dosage.

A Tale of Two Tylenols

If your pediatrician recommends either **Concentrated Tylenol Infants' Drops** or **Children's Tylenol Suspension Liquid** (both acetaminophen), pay special attention to which product you're using and what the dose is—and, as always, *use only the dispenser that's made for that product*. The Infants' Drops are much more concentrated than the Children's Tylenol Suspension Liquid, even though most parents assume—wrongly—that the drops are weaker. The Infants' Drops come with (guess what?) a little dropper for dispensing, while the children's liquid comes with a little cup. Don't mix up the meds or the dispensers. The perils of confusing them: The Institute for Safe Medication Practices reported that one parent was about to give her twenty-seven-month-old two *teaspoons* (or about ten milliliters) of the infant drops instead of two droppers (1.6 mililiters) because she didn't realize the drops were much more concentrated. Luckily, she called her pharmacist beforehand and didn't make the mistake. This example points out why it's so important to read instructions carefully—and to proceed slowly and cautiously when using over-the-counter meds.

What's in Dr. Jen's Medicine Cabinet?

- **Acetaminophen and ibuprofen** (Children's Tylenol and Motrin)—they're my go-to pain relievers and fever reducers. I usually turn to ibuprofen first because taste matters with kids, especially *my* kids, and when I try to give them acetaminophen, most of it ends up on the floor or on their pajamas, not in their tummies. I'm sure you can relate!
- **Antihistamines** such as Benadryl (diphenhydramine), Claritin (loratadine), and Zyrtec (cetirizine), for allergic reactions and hives. Thankfully, most antihistamines are now available in oral disintegrating tablets, which are amazing—they dissolve so quickly that kids don't have time to spit them out.
- **An antibiotic ointment,** such as Neosporin, for cuts and scrapes.
- **Saline drops** for stuffy congested noses.
- **Moisturizers,** such as Cetaphil, Lubriderm, and Aquaphor, to prevent/relieve dry itchy skin and chapped lips.
- **Honey,** because studies show that it's a more effective cough suppressant than many over-the-counter remedies. However, *never* give honey to children younger than twelve months due to the risk of infant botulism (see top of page 24).

* * * * * * * * * * * * * * * * * * *

Infant botulism: An illness caused by certain bacteria spores found in soil, air, dust, and some foods, including honey. While rare (about a hundred cases per year in the U.S.), left untreated it can cause paralysis or fatality in infants, whose gastrointestinal tracts aren't fully developed. Older children and adults don't have problems with honey.

* * * * * * * * * * * * * * * * * * *

What's Your Pharmacist's First Name?

Joan? Mike? Ariel? José? Siew Lee? If you don't know, you should. Pharmacists are valuable pals. (Here's a shout-out to Charles at Cherry's Pharmacy on East Sixty-sixth Street!) If there's a group of people a parent really needs to get up close and friendly with, it's your local pharmacy staff. Sure, workers rotate, hours change, and the person who knows you might not be there every time you stop by. But most pharmacies try to keep regular staff so that customers can develop some familiarity with them. Nonchain neighborhood pharmacies are a great resource. They're usually privately owned and can offer personal attention that the chains often cannot. If there's a pharmacist who specializes in children's medications, he will be able to formulate meds into suspensions (liquid forms of medicines that normally come in pills) *and* add extra flavoring to make the meds taste better. Some pharmacies even offer a choice of flavors—almost like ice cream. Trust me, flavored meds are miraculous for fussy kids who won't take plain medicine!

Make good use of the pharmacy's "consultation" window, which gives you a little privacy and some one-on-one time with the pharmacist. You can also call and ask to speak to the pharmacist if you want to double-check whether, for example, combining Tylenol (acetaminophen) with Benadryl (diphenhydramine) is okay for your child. If you do call, make sure the pharmacist pulls up your child's prescription record and checks any other meds your child might be taking. Don't forget to mention vitamins and herbals, too. And please don't ever feel like you're wasting the pharmacist's time by asking good questions and double-checking medications. Pharmacists, like docs, are busy people, but it's their job to be there for you and to answer questions.

You can also ask the pharmacist to print out extra information if you have any concerns. Pharmacists have access to a lot of medication details.

When you pick up a prescription, compare the pill or liquid to the patient information leaflet stapled to the pharmacy bag—often, it will have a small picture of the pill or medicine. Make sure they match. If not, ask the pharmacist or technician to reconfirm the order. It's possible that your doctor ordered a generic medication that looks different, but ask anyway. And as with all health care staff, ask nicely and be appreciative. When was the last time someone thanked you for being a super mom or dad?

What Not to Mix

When your child swallows a pill or takes a liquid med, it lands in the stomach with whatever else he's eaten, including that handful of dirt from the backyard. The dirt may be fine, but certain foods don't mix with certain drugs. The combination can change how well the medication works or even cause a serious reaction. When getting a prescription, always ask your pediatrician and pharmacist about potential food interactions, and read the package insert.

DON'T MIX THIS DRUG ...	WITH THIS FOOD ...	BECAUSE ...
Theophylline (an asthma medication)	Caffeine (in many sodas, chocolate, tea)	The combo can cause nausea, heart palpitations, or seizures
Erhthromycin	Grapefruit juice	Grapefruit juice increases the drug's absorption
Tetracycline (an antibiotic rarely given to kids under eight because it can stain teeth)	Any food or milk	They can decrease the drug's effectiveness
Ritalin	Foods or drinks with caffeine or decongestants	They can increase blood pressure and tachycardia and heart arrhythmias

Tips for Getting the Medicine Down

Few things can be as challenging as trying to get a pill or dropper full of liquid into a squirming tot's mouth. (Okay, maybe getting them into an angry cat's mouth.) But both get easier with practice. I've given meds to babies about twenty-five thousand times, so I can do it with the ease of a headwaiter uncorking a Chardonnay. I'm happy to share my hard-won tips.

Infants: Tag-team them. Have one person give the medicine

26

while the other holds the infant, wrapped in a blanket to keep flailing arms at bay. Try this technique: Using a dropper, squirt in the medication slowly toward the side and back of the cheek. If your baby vomits within twenty minutes of taking the medicine, call your pediatrician. Another dose may be necessary.

Toddlers: Pretend to give a dose of medicine to your child's favorite stuffed animal or doll first. That sometimes works. Or freeze your child's taste buds with a Popsicle before giving the medicine. Distraction works well, too, since toddlers have a short attention span. Try giving the medicine while your child is watching a movie or being read to. If all else fails, try the tag-team method, above. Usually, after you get a few doses down, a toddler will realize that there's no avoiding the medicine and give in.

Kids: They often want to be in control, so let them hold the dispenser. (Just make sure to supervise.) Often another form can be substituted for medication that comes in pills—a liquid, a chewable form, or an "instant" dissolving tab that can be placed right on the tongue. If there's not an alternative form, sometimes pills can be crushed and added to applesauce or another soft food—but check on that first as it could alter the med's effectiveness.

Allergies and Reactions: What's the Diff?

While the terms are used interchangeably, a true allergic reaction to a medication usually involves hives, wheezing, or difficulty swallowing or breathing (all can be a true emergency). Your child may have a nonallergic reaction or side effect that may include stomachache, diarrhea, or sun sensitivity. Side effects do not necessarily mean that your child should stop taking the medicine, but call your doctor right away and check if you suspect something is wrong.

Most reactions are not serious. Since kids are typically taking

Have a Problem? Report It! Now!

In addition to telling your doctor when your child reacts to a medicine, you should also report it to the FDA if your child has a serious or unusual reaction. The FDA has a program called MedWatch for reporting serious reactions and problems with medications. If enough children have the same reaction to a medicine, it will be investigated, so it's really important to take this step and report it. For more information, go to www.fda.gov/medwatch/.

only one medication at a time for an acute condition (such as an ear infection), we don't have to worry quite as much as we do for adults, who might be taking several medications at once, which can complicate things.

If your child breaks out in hives, for example, call the doctor, who'll advise you what to do next, such as stop the medicine or switch to something else. Your doctor will note the reaction in your child's medical record so that the medication won't be prescribed again. Add this to your home records, too, and tell the pharmacist so the reaction is in your child's prescription record.

The chance of a reaction is worrisome, I know, but the benefits of a needed medication usually far outweigh the possible side effects.

Childproof? Don't Bet on It

I doubt I have to tell you that calling any container "childproof" is a misnomer. I've seen kids as young as eighteen months who can pry open vials of meds, and plenty of adults who can't. By age three, some children are *very* skilled at popping open "child-resistant" tops. So please make sure to keep all meds, prescription or not, out of sight and out of reach, preferably in locked places. Be sure that when Grandma and Grandpa come to stay that they secure their meds too. Many kids get into trouble when medications are left on a counter after use. Also, try to keep tabs on about how many pills are in your own medication bottles. If your child gets into one of them, it helps to know about how many pills he took.

Keep vitamins out of reach too. Formulas that contain iron are said to be responsible for 30 percent of children's deaths from poisoning. That's why you should never tell kids that vitamins are "candy." When Mom or Dad's not looking, they may grab more candy. Say, five or six handfuls. It doesn't help that a lot of kids' vitamins are shaped like cartoon characters and come in fun bottles. It makes it easier to get kids to take their vitamins—but don't make it easy for kids to try to take them themselves.

Also, make sure your child's younger siblings don't try to imitate a big brother or sister who takes a med. You may be able to trust your nine-year-old to take his medication after he finishes a video game, but you can't trust his two-year-old sister not to swipe his waiting pill off the kitchen table. An estimated 53,500 children, ages four and under, are treated in emergency departments every year after swallowing medicines that weren't intended for them.

Smart Storage for Fragile Meds

You know to store meds in a safe place so you protect your children, but what about protecting the meds? They need some love, too (as if the $50 copay weren't enough). The bathroom medicine cabinet is the worst place to keep medication. The humidity and warmth can break down the formulations, rendering them ineffective. Heat and light can weaken them, too. A great place for medications is on the top shelf of a dark, cool linen closet. A high kitchen cabinet (one that's *not* above the stove or refrigerator) is another possibility. But don't forget that some enterprising tykes like to push chairs over to kitchen counters and climb.

Don't Just Trash Them!

Refrain from throwing medications into the kitchen or bathroom trash. *Please.* Young children and pets can find and eat them. Also, do not flush medicines down the toilet. Yes, I know this was the standard advice for decades but recent studies have found that medicines disposed of in sewer and septic systems can seep into the environment. (That's right, there may be a teeny bit of cholesterol medication in your tap water.) The FDA recommends taking unused, unneeded, or expired medicines out of their containers, mixing them with coffee grounds or kitty litter, and then putting that in a sealed bag or empty can. That will keep kids and pets from accidentally getting into the medicine. Some communities have a waste program where you can bring old meds for safe disposal. Ask your pharmacist about this or check www.smarxtdisposal.net.

Preventing Medication Errors at Home

Follow these commandments to help protect your baby, toddler, or child from medication mishaps by your own hand.

❑ **Don't buy over-the-counter medicines that promise "multi-symptom relief."** It's best if you give your child, for example, a simple pain reliever with only one active ingredient rather than something with several different kinds of medicines. Why? Four reasons: (1) If you use a multisymptom product, you'll probably give your child medicines he doesn't need. (2) I've found that multi-ingredient products often undertreat fever or pain, or overdo the decongestant, which makes the child jittery. (3) Many "multi" products contain acetaminophen, but if you don't realize that and give your child an additional dose of Tylenol (acetaminophen), you risk an overdose. Read labels! (4) Finally, if your child reacts to a multisymptom medication, how will you know which ingredient was the culprit? Keep it simple: Stick with single-action meds.

❏ **Don't give children medicines that contain aspirin-like compounds.** By now, you know not to give kids sixteen or younger aspirin because of its connection in kids to Reye's syndrome, which can cause brain and liver damage. But did you know that there are aspirin-like ingredients (called salicylates) in other medications? One example is Kaopectate (bismuth subsalicylate), which should not be taken by children. Adult-strength Pepto-Bismol, used to settle an upset stomach, also contains bismuth subsalicylate, which isn't good for kids; however, Pepto-Bismol children's chewable tablets contain calcium carbonate, which is okay for kids to take. (Double-check that you're using *Children's* Pepto chewables, though, because there are adult chewables, too.) So again, make sure to read labels and/or check with your pediatrician or pharmacist if you're not 100 percent *sure* a medication is safe for your child.

Reye's syndrome: A disease that can affect all organs of the body and may be fatal. Symptoms include nausea, vomiting, rapid breathing, and behavioral changes.

❏ **Avoid decongestants.** They are usually given for a stuffy nose, but they contain ingredients that can actually make your child agitated, irritable, or unable to sleep. Instead, try saline nose drops before bedtime or use a cool-mist humidifier or a warm

bath or shower to help your kid breathe easier during the
night.

❑ **Remember to "shake well before using."** When a liquid
med says this, do it. Many, *many* parents don't shake well, if
at all—and that may mean your child gets either a too-weak
dose (because the powerful stuff has settled to the bottom) or
a too-strong one (because the potent ingredients have risen to
the top). Either way, not good. Not to mention a big waste of
time and money.

❑ **Check the expiration date.** You know most drugs only last a
year, right? Sometimes even less. That's why they're stamped
with expiration dates. In some cases, drugs actually become
more potent if they are used past the safe date, but more often
they lose their effectiveness. Regardless, if the date is up, toss
'em. Take five minutes right now to go through any old con-

Are Depression Meds Linked to Suicide?

 Does using selective serotonin reuptake inhibitors
(SSRIs) to treat major depression boost a teen's
risk of suicide?

No. Adolescents with major depression are seven times
more likely to commit suicide than those not suffering
from major depression. Treating the depression helps to
prevent suicide. However, parents should know that taking an SSRI may increase suicidal thinking (by twofold),
but it does not increase the risk of suicide.

If psychiatric medicines are prescribed for your
child, it is extremely important for him to be monitored
closely by his doctor.

tainers of pills, check expiration dates, and purge the old stuff. (See page 30 for the best way to get rid of old meds.)

❏ **Don't share prescription medications with your kids, relatives, or friends.** Yes, we should all learn to share. But when it comes to pharmaceuticals, selfish is in. *Never give your child another person's medicine.* I know how expensive drugs are, but this practice can be fatal. Your children may have different symptoms or reactions to the med. Certainly, few children weigh exactly the same amount, which is what the dose for the prescription will be based on. Big problems can result. It's much less hassle to make another trip to the doctor's office than to the emergency department. And much cheaper. And *much* safer.

Medications and Hospital or Emergency Department Visits

In chapters 5 and 6, I discuss the importance of knowing what drugs have been prescribed to your child—including the correct dosages, concentrations, and how often they're taken—during a hospital or emergency department visit. Although doctors and nurses do take precautions to prevent medication errors, your diligence can be a safety net to *ensure* that these errors don't happen to your child.

CHAPTER 1 POP QUIZ ANSWERS

1. When is it okay to give your baby or young child baby aspirin? The answer is C: never, ever! (page 19)

2. Which of these ailments should be treated with antibiotics? The answer is D: none of them! All are caused by viruses, so taking antibiotics would be useless—and would contribute to an impending medical crisis. (page 11)

3. What has been shown to be more effective than many over-the-counter cough suppressants? The answer is C—but only for kids older than one. Never give honey to kids younger than one. (page 23)

4. Determining the correct dose of medication for a child is usually based on . . . The answer is A, weight in kilograms. (page 14)

5. What's the disturbing little "secret" that often makes giving a child even a well-known drug somewhat risky? The answer is C—thousands of drugs that are given to kids haven't been tested on children. (page 5)

6. What is the best way to dispose of unneeded medications? The answer is C. Though I wouldn't be surprised if D becomes the new advice by next year. (page 30)

Chapter 2

How Do You
Find Dr. Right?

How Smart Parents Locate Smart Pediatricians

POP QUIZ

Have you made a love connection with a pediatrician? Or are you unhappy with your child's doc? Or are you just starting to look for one? Take this quiz to find out if your search for a pediatrician is on the right track. If you can correctly answer the following questions (there may be more than one correct answer), feel free to skip to the next chapter. But if you miss a question or two, read on. (Answers can be found at the end of the chapter.)

1. When shopping for a pediatrician, what should you always ask the pediatrician's office manager?
   A. How many children of other doctors does this pediatrician treat?
   B. Does this pediatrician hate middle-of-the-night calls from parents a little more or a little less than the average pediatrician?
   C. If this is a group practice, which doctor would the office manager call in an emergency?
   D. All of the above
   E. A and C

2. A parent who's tempted to call an ambulance every time her child skins a knee would probably be best served by a pediatrician whose treatment style . . .
    A. Mirrors the parent's, so each and every concern is examined and treated immediately
    B. Complements the parent's by being more relaxed with a "watch and wait" approach

3. How long is too long to regularly wait in a pediatrician's waiting room?
    A. Ten minutes
    B. Twenty to thirty minutes
    C. Forty-five minutes
    D. Until every parent and child who entered after you has been seen

4. Even in a pinch, you should *not* use a retail health clinic (often found in pharmacies) to treat your child for . . .
    A. Rashes, poison ivy, bug bites, hives, or severe sunburn
    B. Strep throat symptoms (requiring a culture test for strep throat)
    C. Breathing difficulty
    D. Cuts or bruises that don't require stitches
    E. Swimmer's ear

5. Never tell your child that a shot . . .
    A. Will hurt
    B. Will be given to them if they keep misbehaving
    C. Is absolutely necessary
    D. Will be followed by a trip to the mall and a new toy

6. Which of these is something many pediatricians consider a time-wasting pet peeve?
    A. Doorknob moments
    B. Helicopter parenting
    C. "I forgot my checkbook"

7. What is *not* a legitimate reason to give your pediatrician the boot?
  A. Not calling you back within sixty minutes after office hours, on more than one occasion
  B. Refusing to prescribe an antibiotic for your child, even though you were sure it was necessary
  C. Using expired vaccines
  D. Being of little help during an emergency situation

Two weeks ago, I saw a seven-year-old girl with a severe ear infection. Her mother had found me on the Mount Sinai Physician Referral Hotline that morning.

"We love our regular pediatrician, but she doesn't work on Wednesdays," she explained.

Happy to be able to help but also curious, I asked, "Not a big fan of anyone on her backup team?"

"She doesn't have a backup team," the parent replied.

Now, this woman seemed like a typical mom. I doubt she let her daughter play on an interstate highway or with matches. But when it came to picking her baby's doctor, she wasn't at her brightest. If her daughter had a serious medical problem on a Wednesday, or whenever this pediatrician was unavailable, the girl would have to be treated by a doctor who knew nothing about her. A similar situation for you and your child could make a difference in how your child is cared for in critical moments, which is why choosing the right pediatrician is one of the most important decisions you'll ever make as a parent.

"Eenie, Meenie, Minie..."

I was pretty lucky when I went through this particular rite of passage. When my husband David and I had our first child thirteen years ago, I knew just the right pediatrician for us. No, it wasn't me. Although I'm fortunate enough to be the right pediatrician for many patients, I knew I couldn't be objective as Dr. Mom. But I had watched the right doctor for my kids for several years. I knew her reputation in our professional circles—where flaws aren't sugarcoated. And I had the advantage of being able to compare her skills and decisions with those of many pediatricians, including myself. I knew how this physician thought, how she reacted in emergencies, and how well she recognized her limits. Most parents don't have all of these advantages, but they do have far more than they think.

Nevertheless, many parents select their doctor based on two things: If the practice accepts their insurance, and if the office is within a twenty-minute drive. Sure, many people ask their friends, their family members, and their own docs for recommendations, and others do a few Internet searches to see if likely pediatricians have won any awards or perhaps have a police record. Some also ask good basic questions: "Are you affiliated with a teaching hospital? Are you board certified in pediatrics?" (See page 56 for more on board certification.)

All are good steps to take, but they could lead to dozens of pediatricians who are good doctors but not necessarily the *right* doctors.

So how can you find the *right* doctor?

Smart Shoppers Already Know the Drill

Let's say I'm in the market for a new hairstylist—someone I can trust with my appearance and see happily every few weeks for years. Being around the corner isn't going to seal the deal.

I will shop around and ask my friends, family, even someone in the grocery line who's got a great haircut for recommendations. I might try out a few by getting a basic trim, or—less of a commitment—by getting an updo or blow-dry (no scissors!). If I'm not happy with the results and the person, I'll move on until I find exactly the right fit for me.

Now, you've probably invested that kind of time in some sort of search. If it wasn't choosing a stylist, perhaps it was picking out a stroller or a paint color or a preschool—or even a pair of jeans or a flat-panel TV. Finding a pediatrician shouldn't be much different. The same or greater diligence you'd put into any of those searches should go into finding the right doctor for your child.

So let's lay out a plan.

Pediatricians Do More than Prescribe Meds and Give Shots

 Your pediatrician does many jobs, but in general you can expect the doctor to:

* Monitor your child's growth and development
* Diagnose, treat, and explain illnesses and treatments
* Provide referrals to other specialists and work with them when needed
* Help with a potpourri of other issues: exercise and nutrition, toilet training and bedwetting, learning disabilities, emotional and behavioral problems, and dealing with death, separation, and divorce, or any other major life changes that may affect your child

Basically, you should view me (I'm standing in for your pediatrician here) as a partner whose main goal is to keep your child physically and mentally healthy.

When to Start Searching

Like any important project, searching for a great pediatrician is less daunting when you break it into small tasks and spread them out over time. **If you are pregnant,** start looking at least three months before you're due. This allows plenty of time to find the child doctor of your dreams. **If you already have a new baby** but don't have a regular pediatrician yet, start now so that you, your baby, and your future pediatrician have the advantage of starting a relationship as early as possible.

If you already have a pediatrician, that's fantastic. But if you have any niggling concerns, this chapter will help you decide if that doctor is indeed right for your children and for *you*. You'll either feel more confident about your choice or realize you need to press the "eject" button and find someone else.

Start by Networking

First, get recommendations for pediatricians from the most obvious sources: your obstetrician or nurse midwife, and your own primary care doctor. If you're adopting, which brings special concerns (see page 59), you can also ask the adoption agency for recommendations. Then ask friends, family, coworkers, and neighbors. Getting word-of-mouth referrals from people you trust is incredibly important (it's how I get most of my patients). It's like getting the name of a good caterer from a neighbor or an aunt—except, of course, a caterer won't be meeting your child in an emergency department at four A.M.

When you're asking someone for a doctor recommendation, include some or all of these questions in your friendly grilling:

- Why do you like this particular pediatrician?
- How long has this doc treated your child (or children)?
- What's the usual wait time in the office before an appointment?

- What is the office staff like?
- In an emergency, have you found the doctor to be highly accessible, either by phone or in person?

If the same one or two names keep coming up, great. Put those doctors at the top of your list. But don't discard the others yet. There's always the *teeny* chance that some of the people who give you enthusiastic recommendations 1) are satisfied with mediocre health care; or 2) have been lucky recipients of sporadic good treatment from a doctor who disappoints many other patients. You're just gathering information now, so throw all possible candidates into the pool.

Have Some Great Candidates?

When you have at least a few names, it's time to narrow down your list.

Let's start with one of the biggest issues: **money.** Check your insurance plan to find out which pediatricians, if any, are in your insurer's provider network. If your health insurer only covers in-network doctors, these contenders just got some stars by their names. If your insurer covers a percentage of the expenses for out-of-network docs, see "Can Going 'Out-of-Network' Work for You?" on page 42.

Next, check out these doctors online. Start with an ordinary Google search. You may find a hospital bio page for the doctor . . . or, oops, a page on a social-networking site with wild photos of the doc in Cancún on spring break. Some general searches can also quickly give you an idea if the doctor has authored any clinical studies (good sign) or worked with local organizations (also good). Next, check the site of the American Board of Medical Specialties (www.abms.org) to be certain that candidates are board certified in specialties that focus on the care of children, such as pediatrics or family medicine. See "What

---

Can Going "Out-of-Network" Work for You?

Having health insurance that only covers "in-network" doctors can really limit your options. You'll either have to choose a pediatrician from their in-network list or foot every bill yourself—and for most people, that's not an option. However, many insurance plans will cover a percentage of the cost of a doctor who's not in their network. If your dream doc isn't, and you can afford the extra fees for an out-of-network doctor, it may be the right choice for you and your child.

Kind of Primary Care Provider Do You Need?" (pages 56–57) for more good choices. The ABMS site can also provide you with additional candidates if your list is thin.

Any Skeletons in the Closet?

Other than the one used for demonstration purposes, that is. Find out if your candidates have any nasty incidents lurking in their past. While a cursory search won't reveal everything, check the Federation of State Medical Boards (FSMB) to see if there have been any serious disciplinary actions or professional peer reviews (trouble brewing) against the pediatrician. This is rare, but I'd sure want to know about it. In most states, the information is public and free. Find your state's link at www.fsmb.org/directory_smb.html or call (817) 868-4000 to get the number for your state board.

Time for a Meet-and-Greet

Okay, time to call the candidates and schedule a "meet-and-greet"—a prenatal or preadoption consultation, or a consultation to switch from Dr. So-So to Dr. Right. Most insurance companies don't cover this kind of visit, even though it's necessary, but—good news—many physicians welcome these interviews and don't charge for them. Still, some do. Ask when you call for an appointment.

If at all possible, bring your child along so you can see how the doc and the staff interact with her. Arrive early so you can do some stealth detective work. Look around.

- Is the waiting room empty or chock-full of parents and sick, crabby kids? Neither is a great sign—unless you're visiting at seven A.M. or plunk in the middle of cold and flu season.
- Is the place clean? (Don't forget to check the restroom; grime is a big warning sign.)
- Is the office staff polite and friendly or surly and dismissive? Did they make you and your little one feel welcome?
- Does the office appear organized, or does it look like they use pitchforks to stack the file folders?
- Is the waiting area kid-friendly, with dancing-bear wall decals and lots of books, toys, and games? Or is it as bleak as a police precinct?
- Do the toys look clean and in good shape, or are they grimy and shabby?
- Can you see yourself coming here with your child?

Chat up the other parents and ask if they're happy with the pediatrician; if it's a group practice, ask which docs they do and *don't* like. Are the waits long? (Half an hour should be the longest.) Is getting a return call from the pediatrician difficult? Is the staff helpful when there's an insurance snafu?

TIP: Bring your own toys! When I take my kids to the pediatrician, I always bring a couple of favorite toys from home for them to play with, especially during cold and flu season, when the office toys are likely to be germ riddled. At my office, we wash the toys regularly and disinfect them with Lysol, and we also give parents disinfectant wipes to clean toys before their kids dive in. But there's no getting around it: Lots of sick kids touch those toys, and we can't clean them every fifteen seconds. Quite often, at the very second a parent is ripping open a disinfectant wipe, his three-year-old is across the room clutching the truck that a two-year-old licked a minute ago. Smart parents bring their own toys. Bringing your own toys also means that they can be brought into the exam room to keep your child entertained.

Even if you're disappointed before you even see the pediatrician, don't leave yet. Just like a job interview, it's worth doing, even if only for the experience.

Schmooze the Office Manager

During your visit, always—*always*—seek out that treasure trove of information who resides near the waiting room. Yes, the office manager. The person who knows many things. Good things and bad things. Charm some key intelligence out of this oracle. Start with small talk, throw in a genuine compliment ("Nice earrings!"), then ask the insider questions that follow. (Make a copy of them to use as a cheat sheet.)

Questions for the Office Manager

☐ **"Do you or any of your family members use this pediatrician?"** If not, gently probe as to why.

☐ **"How many children of *physicians* does the doctor treat?"** Twenty? Thirty? If it's two, then my kid wouldn't be the third. This can depend on your geographic area, of course. Pediatricians who work in regions that have few physicians may treat relatively few children of other doctors. But in general I'd strongly prefer a pediatrician who has the trust of other MDs.

☐ **"What are your office hours? Do you have early morning, evening, and weekend hours to accommodate working parents or emergency situations?"**

☐ **"How much vacation does the doctor take every year?"** If it's more than one month, hesitate. You instinctively know that your kid's emergency will happen when "The Doctor Is Out." I know pediatricians who take four months of vacation a year, so definitely check this out!

☐ **"Last year, how many conferences did the doctor go to? How many continuing medical education courses did she take?"** The office manager likely processes the paperwork for conferences and courses. If the response is "Zero," that's a bad answer. However, ask the doctor the same question directly. Many continuing-education courses are done online now, so it's possible the doc has taken courses the office manager doesn't know a thing about.

☐ "Have you ever seen the pediatrician respond to an emergency situation? Did he take control? Was he as effective as he could have been?" Ask if the doctor is typically stoic and calm in emergencies or excited and tense. Calm is better.

☐ "Speaking of emergencies, in a life-or-death situation, which pediatrician in this practice would you ideally want to treat your child? Why?" If she doesn't pick the doctor you're principally interested in, you have more homework to do. Tip: The office manager may answer tactfully or cryptically, so read between the lines. If she says, "They're all great . . . honestly, I'd feel comfortable with Dr. Jones, or any of the partners," that means "Dr. Jones."

☐ "Compared with other pediatricians you've worked with, how does this doctor feel about getting phone calls at home? Does it bother her a little more than the rest or a little less?" You're really hoping for a superlative response here, like "She doesn't mind at all." Something more tepid, along the lines of "She's not crazy about after-hours calls," can be a telling answer.

☐ "Compared with other pediatricians you've worked with, is this doctor a bit anal about keeping charts and things well organized or a little more relaxed about that stuff than the others?" You definitely want anal. (Though you don't necessarily have to express that to the office manager.)

☐ "How does the doctor treat the office staff?" Meaning the nurses, receptionists, clerical helpers, and the office manager, not just other docs in the practice. Ask if "please" and "thank you" are common, or is yelling more typical? If the office manager does some polite eye rolling or gives evasive answers, there's a good chance that the doc is, um, a bit of a bully. Politeness may not always trump exceptional skill or talent, but it can be critical in fostering a good relationship with patients and parents. It's one thing if a world-class specialist that you'll only have to deal with once is a terror, but for your day-to-day pediatrician? I think niceness counts big-time. You don't want to hesitate phoning the doc in an iffy situation because you're worried about somebody's bad attitude.

Now Grill the Doctor

After your incredibly fruitful time in the waiting room—which hopefully was not excessively long—you'll be ushered back to interview the candidate. Here's a checklist of questions I would recommend asking; add any others you like.

Questions for a New Pediatrician

Start with getting basic credentials and some personal info.

☐ How long have you been practicing? How long have you been in this office?

☐ Do you have children? If so, who's their doctor? (Being a parent can help a doctor be a better pediatrician, so you might give bonus points for docs who have kids.)

☐ What medical school did you attend? Do you have any special medical interests? Do you have any specializations?

☐ How long have you been board certified in pediatrics or family medicine? Do you have a lifelong certification or do you periodically take recertifying exams?

☐ Are you currently board certified in something in addition to pediatrics or family medicine?

☐ Which hospital(s) are you affiliated with? (This could be a deal breaker if it's not a hospital you've picked—see chapter 6.)

☐ Does that hospital have a pediatric floor or wing? Is it staffed with pediatric residents for twenty-four-hour care? Is it equipped to handle pediatric emergencies? Is the hospital accredited by The Joint Commission?

The Joint Commission

The Joint Commission, a private, not-for-profit organization, has been the nation's leader in continuously improving patient safety and health care quality for almost sixty years. The Joint Commission is the principal standards setter and evaluator for a variety of health care organizations, including hospitals, ambulatory care, behavioral health care, home care, laboratories, and long-term care. Joint Commission accreditation—the coveted Gold Seal of Approval™— means that a health care organization complies with the most rigorous standards of performance. More information about The Joint Commission can be found in later chapters or by visiting its website at www.jointcommission.org.

Next, determine how well the pediatrician handles emergencies.

- [ ] During an emergency, how do you prefer your patients to coordinate with you?
- [ ] How do you handle late-night calls and emergencies?
- [ ] Can I have your cell phone number for true emergencies?
- [ ] Will you come to the ER? (If this question begets laughter, consider that a big check in the "Keep Hunting" column.)
- [ ] Will you visit my child if he or she is hospitalized? Will you continue to be the primary care coordinator if my child is in the hospital?

Next, ask about the pediatrician's treatment experience, philosophies, and patients.

☐ How many patients do you see on a weekly basis?

☐ What is your viewpoint on breastfeeding? (You need only ask this if you're seeking a pediatrician before your baby's birth or looking for a new pediatrician while you're still breastfeeding.)

☐ What is your experience with children who have special needs (such as autism, ADHD, or cerebral palsy)? Ask this even if your children don't have special needs. In my opinion, pediatricians with intense experience in treating special-needs children typically have greater patience and more finely tuned skills of perception.

☐ What is your experience in treating adopted children and dealing with cultural issues? (Only ask this if it's relevant to your child.)

☐ What is your perspective on antibiotics and immunizations? (If the pediatrician's viewpoints differ markedly from yours or from the mainstream—see pages 97 and 262—ask why.)

☐ Add specific questions that are relevant to your child, including ones about diet and exercise issues if your child is overweight.

Next, find out how easy it will be to deal with this doctor for routine stuff.

- ☐ Do you leave room in your schedule for same-day sick appointments?

- ☐ Is this a group practice? If not, who fills in for you when you're unavailable? (The more doctors in the practice, the more likely you'll have good backup if your doctor isn't available in an emergency.)

- ☐ How do you handle phone calls? Do you have a special time set aside for parents to call with questions? If not, how long should I expect to wait to hear from you?

- ☐ Do you do any quick lab tests in your office, or is all lab work sent to an outside lab? How long does it take to get results? (It's ideal if your pediatrician does some rapid tests, such as strep throat cultures, right in the office; it saves time and hassle.)

- ☐ What is your e-mail policy? Can I send you general health questions by e-mail? What about questions if my child is sick? How quickly do you tend to reply to e-mails? Is there a fee for e-mail correspondence? (Generally, pediatricians don't charge for this, but make sure.)

Finally, it's time to talk money. You can also get this info from the office staff, but if you have special concerns, speak directly to the doctor.

☐ What are your fees? Do you have a list of them broken down by service?

☐ What are your payment policies? Which insurance plans do you participate in? Do you file insurance claims or do I?

☐ Do you charge fees to fill out forms or send copies of charts? (Pediatricians typically send out several forms per child per year to schools, after-school programs, camps, etc. Make sure any fees for this don't come as a nasty surprise.)

Grade That Pediatrician

For your eyes only.

☐ Did the doctor make you and your child feel comfortable?

☐ Did the doctor explain things well? If your child is old enough to know what's going on, did the doc explain things at a level that your child can understand and talk directly to your child?

☐ Did the doctor listen to questions and concerns or seem rushed?

☐ Do you share similar philosophies on child-rearing issues such as breastfeeding, circumcision, sleep problems, diet, and exercise?

Did You Make a Love Connection?

I hope so. But if you visited only one pediatrician, be skeptical about love at first sight; interview at least two more to be sure you're going with the right person. The chemistry you felt with the doctor is just as important as the answers you got to your questions. Did you like the doc's style? Did anything put you off? If you felt at all intimidated or talked down to, this may not be a match. If you felt rushed or just didn't click with the pediatrician's personality, you may not want to go forward either. A lot of people have a gut feeling when they find the right pediatrician, so listen to your inner voice.

You Be the Judge

Finally, make sure you are comfortable with the doctor's age and gender. With a little luck, you and your children will be relying on this person's medical care and advice for twenty years or more. Do you want to fall in love with a pediatrician who's hitting retirement in five years? If your kids are in their teens, maybe. But if you've got an infant, you might want to think twice.

During the first year of your baby's life, you will visit the pediatrician a dozen times—and that's just for vaccinations and wellness checks. That doesn't include ear infections, coughs, colds, or mishaps. You'd better be able to work well with this person and be thinking about the future. If you have a boy, you might prefer a male pediatrician so your son feels comfortable as he grows, especially through puberty. (Yes, your little angel will go through puberty someday.) If you have a girl, you might prefer a female pediatrician for the same reasons. (At least there are options now!)

When I chose a pediatrician for my children, I wanted a female who'd had kids herself. I know that I tend to relate to this type of physician best . . . perhaps because we share the same experiences. But those are *my* preferences. Bottom line: Pick someone who suits *your* preferences. It's okay to be persnickety.

Do Your Styles Sync?

Even if the doc seems smart, kind, and trustworthy, try to get a handle on whether his or her medical style complements yours. For instance, if you are a chronic over-the-top worrier—someone who inwardly considers calling 911 every time your child skins a knee—you may want a doctor who exudes calm and takes a "watch-and-wait" approach (as well as one who's skilled at talking worried parents off the ledge). However, if you tend to be the watch-and-wait type yourself, you may want a doctor with a more gung-ho, proactive treatment style who will give more intense scrutiny to symptoms you might minimize. Make sure you see eye to eye when it comes to how the doctor views your role. Does the doctor look at parents as partners or prefer to be the Lone Ranger? Make sure you both have the same expectations. Also, you need to determine if you're more comfortable with a *patient-centered* or *paternalistic* relationship with your doctor.

I'll explain. There was a time not so long ago when the patient was in the backseat and the doctor drove the proverbial bus—that is, made all the decisions. Most patients went along with this and tended to view MDs as all-knowing.

Today, however, far fewer doctor-patient relationships fit this paternalistic paradigm. People now have access to almost unlimited medical information via the Internet, TV, books, and magazines. While most people still want and need the knowledge and experience doctors bring to the equation, many also want to be part of the health care process. In fact, one study found 86 percent of parents are likely to participate in decision-making with their doctor. But it also found that those who wanted a paternalistic relationship with their physicians were quite happy with doctors who had the same mind-set.

I strongly prefer parents who view our relationship as a partnership. We are in it together. I provide medical expertise and know-how. You offer information that helps me diagnose and treat. And, of course, you make your final decisions with my guidance.

You also help me help your child—for example, by making sure medications are taken or symptoms are treated or a blood test is scheduled. We really do need each other, and that includes deciding on treatments together. It's best if we're both fully invested in the final outcome: good care and good health for your child.

These roles need not be absolute, by the way. You may want to have a patient-centered relationship, but during emergencies you expect your pediatrician to assume a paternalistic role and take charge. Whatever you envision, talk to the doctor about how you see your role. Personally, I feel like if you're involved in the decision-making, you will be happier with the outcomes.

Speaking of Styles . . .

As a doctor and a mom, I know how important it is for my style to complement the styles of my patients' parents. I always give my office number to parents and tell them to call me if they have further questions or forgot to ask something. I want them to know from the get-go that it's okay to call me. There are no silly questions, just questions that parents may not know the answers to. I'm not bothered by questions, and the right pediatrician for your child shouldn't be either.

What Kind of Primary Care Provider Do You Need?

The right doctor for your child doesn't have to be a pediatrician. It may be one of the experts listed below. You need to figure out who will be the best choice for you and your family. Your decision may also depend on the age of your kids and the health care choices where you live. Here's who does what:

Pediatricians focus on kids' physical, emotional, and social health from birth through young adulthood. They work hard to treat health problems, but they work even harder to prevent trouble by making sure kids have immunizations and regular checkups and eat and sleep properly. Pediatricians must complete four years of medical school and three years of pediatric residency. To be board certified, they must pass a written exam given by the American Board of Pediatrics and then be recertified every seven years. To be eligible for license renewal and to care for patients, a pediatrician must also obtain continuing medical education credits. These are designed to keep doctors up-to-date on the latest medical practices and procedures.

Family physicians also have to complete four years of medical school and three years of residency, which often includes training in pediatrics and/or other areas such as internal medicine, orthopedics, and gynecology. Family physicians are qualified to provide basic care for patients of all ages. To be board certified, they must pass a written exam given by the American Board of Family Medicine and then be recertified every seven years. To be eligible for license renewal and to care for patients, a family physician must also obtain continuing medical education credits. These are designed to keep doctors up-to-date on the latest medical practices and procedures. A family physician can see your child from birth through adulthood, but make sure you ask about age policies since some family physicians don't see children younger than a certain age.

Pediatric nurse practitioners (PNPs) have a master's degree in nursing and get special training in performing physical exams, taking medical histories, and making basic diagnoses in children. If PNPs encounter a complicated medical problem, they're trained to consult with the doctor. PNPs are increasingly popular in group practices because they have the knowledge and time to, say, go over a treatment again when the doctor's already seeing the next patient.

You're Being Interviewed Too

"I'm sorry, I'm not able to take your child as a patient due to my current workload, but I can recommend some other pediatricians who might have more open schedules."

A pediatrician who delivers this line may be telling the whole truth. Perhaps they really couldn't wedge another patient into their schedule with a crowbar. Or they might be telling a half-truth . . . they wouldn't wedge *you* into their schedule with a crowbar. Why? Evaluations go both ways, and docs decide whether they can work with you, too. We may realize our treatment style doesn't sync with yours or just sense that the chemistry between us is off. Or you may ring our alarm bell because you . . .

. . . **have changed doctors a dozen times in the last five years.** That's a red flag that you're not going to be satisfied with any medical professional.

. . . **were a problem parent for a pediatrician five towns away.** What, you think we don't talk to each other? If you had a blowup with Dr. Jones, let Dr. Smith know—briefly, accurately, and without casting aspersions on Dr. Jones.

. . . **have been mysteriously cryptic about your child's medical past or refused to provide medical records** (especially records of consultations with specialists). This often means that a parent already has a fixed viewpoint about a particular issue,

---

Pack Rat Permission Granted

Once you've picked your pediatrician, don't throw away that voluminous pile of information you've collected. What if your wonderful doctor moves out of town? Or decides to quit medicine and hike across America? Or what if a few years from now your daughter doesn't want to see a "boy doctor" anymore? Or your insurance changes and excludes your current pediatrician? Hanging on to that info means you won't have to start over from scratch.

---

such as the source of their child's symptoms, and is shopping for an agreeable doctor who will give them the opinion they want to hear and prescribe the treatment they want rather than actually provide independent medical expertise.

. . . **seem like a "headline parent."** See page 260 in chapter 8 for more on this merry phenomenon.

Winning Records

If you haven't started keeping meticulous records of health history and medical care for yourself *and* your child, please consider yourself nudged in that direction. Good family medical records are so vital that they're a recurring theme in this book. If you haven't started keeping them, it's never too late.

The first step I'd recommend is going to the American Academy of Pediatrics (AAP) website and using the Care Notebook you'll find there (www.medicalhomeinfo.org/tools/care_note book.html). The notebook is an organizing tool that will help you become an expert on your child's and family's health care. You can pick and choose from dozens of handy forms that will help you track immunizations, allergy records, doctor appointments, hospital stays, growth patterns, family and medical history, nutrition, insurance providers, and therapists. There's an online tour to walk you through the steps of putting the Care Notebook together. And you'll find the AAP site is super-useful in general.

MEDICAL RECORDS FOR ADOPTED CHILDREN

Adoption is more popular among Americans than ever before. Each year, about 125,000 native-born children are adopted, and another 23,000 or so children are adopted from countries outside the U.S.

If you adopt a child through a U.S. agency, you should receive a complete medical record for your child to share with your pediatrician. Unfortunately, medical records for children adopted from other countries are not always complete or reliable, and usually the only source of information is the agency or orphanage from which you adopted. Nevertheless, try to obtain as much information as possible for your child's medical records.

- First, you want to learn about the birth parents, including their age, height, weight, ethnicity, education (which can impact their health care), and any medical conditions the mother and father had.
- Second, ask what health care the baby has had since birth. Try your best to get immunization records and growth charts.

For more information on medical records for adopted children, check out these resources.

59

www.aap.org/sections/adoption
Web page on adoption and foster care at the American Academy of Pediatrics (AAP) website

www.adoptioncouncil.org
The National Council for Adoption

www.adoption.org/adopt/national-adoption-information-clearinghouse.php
Website of the National Adoption Information Clearinghouse

adoption.state.gov
Website of the State Department with info on international adoptions

www.adoptivefamilies.com
Link to national magazine for families who are planning to adopt or already have adopted children

www.childwelfare.gov
The Child Welfare Information Gateway, which contains info on both adoption and foster children

www.davethomasfoundation.org
Foundation created by Wendy's founder Dave Thomas, who was an adopted child

www.openadoption.org
Website of the American Association of Open Adoption Agencies

Going High-Tech

Electronic health records (EHRs) are here to stay, in part because the federal government wants *everyone* to have an EHR within ten years as a way to reduce medical errors, improve efficiency, and cut health care costs. So if your pediatrician already uses them—roughly 20 percent do at the moment—you might want to get started. Why? As more and more doctors and hospitals move to EHRs, you'll soon be able to say, "Doctor, can you e-mail me my son's lab results?" Not only will you have them quickly and precisely but you can then copy those results into your own electronic records.

Yes, there are privacy concerns, but frankly, that's true of paper records, too. According to a study done by the *Los Angeles Times*, roughly 150 people (doctors, nurses, technicians, billing clerks) have some access to a patient's medical record during a hospitalization. And that doesn't include insurers and other billing companies. That's why there are strict privacy rules designed to make sure health care information is secure—surely you remember those gazillions of HIPAA (Health Insurance Portability and Accountability Act) forms we had to sign back in the late nineties!

Prepping Your Child— and Yourself—for a Visit

The first year or two of your child's life will include regular wellness visits to the pediatrician to check on growth and development, get vaccinations, and just generally make sure everything is going along fine. But little ones have steel-trap memories, so if your toddler equates going to the doctor *only* with getting shots, you may find yourself with some "splaining" to do. ("So *that's* why the nurse often gives the shots," you're thinking. "Now I get it.") Kids need to understand that docs do a lot more than give shots—tell them that we help kids stay healthy and get well. Whether they are going in for a routine exam or because they are injured or sick, you can help quell their fears.

- Explain why you're going. If it's for a "well-child visit," tell your children the doctor wants to make sure they are growing and that healthy kids go to the doctor to be sure they stay that way. They need to know that **going to the doctor is not a punishment for any misbehavior.** Some kids actually believe this. Really. Not only do some parents not dispel this wrong belief, but I've known a few to even use it as a threat. ("If you don't stop throwing the kitten into the bathtub, I'm going to take you to get a shot!") Naturally, this makes me and other pediatricians crazy! I want kids to think of my office as the place with the cool bears on the wall, not where they go to be punished for putting chewing gum in their sibling's hair.
- If your child is ill, explain that the "doctor will help you feel better." Occasionally younger kids feel guilty about being sick, so assure them that the illness isn't caused by anything they did. Say something like "Sometimes children get sick, and we're lucky to have doctors who can find out why and help you get well."
- It's okay to admit to your child that you don't know what's wrong but that you'll all work together with the doctor to find and fix the problem.
- If your child has an embarrassing problem, like bedwetting or head lice, make sure you explain that it's not their fault and that it happens to *many* children. Kids often feel incredibly embarrassed or guilty about things like this, so discuss it in reassuring language and then put on your best "no biggie" attitude.
- Tell your child what to expect. Basically, play doctor with them at home with a toy medical kit. Use a doll or stuffed animal to

show how the doctor will look in the mouth, eyes, and ears, and listen to the heart with a stethoscope. Explain that the doctor may listen to the tummy, tap the knees, look at the feet, and glance at their "private parts" to make sure everything's healthy. Assure your child that you will be there during the entire exam. Don't forget to bring a favorite doll or stuffed animal along. Like me, your pediatrician may even give Mr. Ted E. Bear an exam, too. No charge.

- Speaking of private parts, most kids are taught that no one should touch them *there,* so explain that sometimes their bodies need to be examined everywhere, including there, to keep them well. Please also explain the differences between appropriate and inappropriate touching, even by a doctor, nurse, mom,

It's Just Between Us . . . Unless It's Serious

As kids reach adolescence, they may stop talking to you about certain issues. Boys may prefer to go to the doctor with their dads, and girls with their moms. If you're the one being shunned, your child still loves you. This is normal, and you can rest assured that the shunning will cease when they're old enough to need a big bump in their allowance or to borrow the car keys. When my patients turn twelve, I create a contract with them. I see them first with a parent and then without. This gives tweens and teens a chance to ask and answer my questions free of embarrassment or fear regarding important issues such as sex, alcohol, smoking, and drugs. My patients also know that if they're doing something to physically hurt themselves, or someone else, I have an obligation to tell their parents.

dad, or grandparent, not to mention a friend or stranger. Your pediatrician can give you some pointers on how to go about this if you're not sure.

- Let your child know if a procedure is going to hurt a little or be embarrassing, but be a little vague on the details so that you don't create unneeded fears.
- Watch your language. If you tell your five-year-old that the doctor will need to "take blood," explain that it will only be a teaspoon or two. Some kids worry that *all* their blood will be taken! (I'm not kidding.)

Ten Tips for the Perfect Office Visit

"You need to bring her in." I know you probably don't want to hear those words, but in many cases, I simply can't answer questions without seeing a child. I'll do what I can to save parents a trip to my office, and many cases can be handled over the phone. But not all. Every child is different, and there are nuances and symptoms that I must physically see in order to diagnose and treat the child. During a sick visit—or any visit for any reason, for that matter—use these ten tips to be a smart communicator and to help your child get quicker treatment.

1. **Don't Be Shy.** Bring a list of questions, starting with the most important ones. Don't be shy about checking your list or taking notes. I'll be impressed that you came prepared. (Just wait to fire away until I have the stethoscope out of my ears.)
2. **Sick . . . How Long?** Please write down what the symptoms are and when each one started. The pattern can make it easier to diagnose problems.
3. **Paint Me a Picture.** If your child is taking any medications, bring those along. That includes vitamins, herbals, and over-the-counter remedies.

4. **Doc, Have You Seen That Study on the Web?** It's great when you come in with information you found on the Internet, in a magazine, or elsewhere. Hey, docs love it when you are well-read and actively involved in your child's care. But it's hard for us to evaluate every health tidbit on, say, the Discovery Channel. If you want us to review some bit of info, e-mail it, fax it, or drop it off in advance, so that we have time to check it out before your office visit. At the same time, give pediatricians a little credit for two things: medical school and years of experience. I see a lot of kids every day, and I may have had experiences that the writer of the *USA Today* article you're panicked about does not.

5. **Attention, Please.** Be focused during the visit. Try to leave other children at home with a sitter. Please turn your cell phone off, too. You want our attention and we want yours.

6. **Promptness Pays.** Arrive on time or even early. We don't want to keep anyone waiting, but if half our patients arrive late, well, you can see why we might run late too.

7. **Huh? I Don't Get It.** If you don't understand something, please ask us to explain it again or in simpler language. We try not to get into doctor-speak, but it happens. Rein us in.

8. **A Sketch, Perhaps?** Would a drawing help to explain a problem or procedure? Sometimes kids and parents can relate better to a picture that shows why an ankle hurts, for example, or a stomach doesn't feel right.

9. **Prefer Parents.** If at all possible, a parent—not a nanny or a sitter—should accompany kids on doctor visits. With working parents, I know that's sometimes tough, but sitters and nannies don't always get the information straight. Also, I may have questions they can't answer. (Another reason why it's preferable to find a pediatrician with evening and/or Saturday hours.) If it's not possible for a parent to come, I will call Mom or Dad before the visit to get the child's history and afterward to give a parent any treatment instructions.

10. **Can You Tell Me Again What You Said?** Don't forget to follow up. If you get home and think, "What was that tip about using the inhaler?" call or e-mail to be sure. It doesn't hurt to ask for written explanations or instructions before leaving your doctor's office, either. That way, you'll have all this information in writing before you're out the door. Also, call about test results. No news is *not* necessarily good news.

One Thing Not to Do

Doctors call them "doorknob moments." It's when the visit is wrapping up, we have our hand on the exam room doorknob to leave, and a parent says, "Wait ... do you think Matthew could be vomiting because he fell down the stairs?"

Maybe you're anxious about telling the doctor something so you save it for last. ("I gave him two tablets instead of one ... could that be a problem?") It's understandable. But here's the thing. We need you to be open about everything during the initial discussion so that we don't miss important clues that could change the diagnosis or treatment. Still, if you do remember something at the last minute, don't be afraid to bring it up. We'd rather have the full picture, doorknob moment or not. And here's a tip that might help: Write down your questions and your child's symptoms before you come.

I Don't Want to Go to the Doctor!

It's a sad fact; not all of my patients love seeing me all of the time. I don't take it personally. Sometimes, kids will open up about why they're afraid of going to the doctor, but more often they remain silent and stew privately. Here's what you need to know, even if they don't tell you.

- Kids worry about pain, especially six- to twelve-year-olds when it comes to shots. Remind them that it stings or pinches for only a second.
- Kids are afraid their parents will leave them alone in the examination room. This is more common in children under seven, but it can happen through age twelve. Tell them you will stay with them throughout the visit.
- Like us, children worry about the unknown. Some kids fear that they are really sick and their parents aren't telling them the truth. If they need surgery or hospitalization, some kids equate that with death, especially if someone they loved and knew, like a grandparent, died after being in the hospital. Offer reassurance and tell your child that the doctor and hospital staff will make sure they feel better and get well. (See chapter 7 for more info on getting through a hospital experience.)
- While it's hard for a pediatrician to be as popular with kids as a cartoon superhero, most docs try to make the experience as pleasant as possible. If your pediatrician seems disinterested or doesn't communicate with you or your child well, it may be time for a change.

The Deal on Retail Health Clinics

You've probably seen the drop-in medical centers in big-box stores like Target or Wal-Mart and in drugstore chains like CVS or Walgreens. There are about a thousand of these "convenient care clinics," "mini clinics," or "minute clinics." As a rule, they handle only common ailments and are staffed by physician assistants and nurse practitioners (NPs), who can order tests and write prescriptions. The cost is relatively low, at about $50 to $75 a visit (or an insurance copay), and the wait is not long. No wonder the clinics are popular with the young and uninsured. Less than half of those who use the clinics have a primary care doctor, which means they serve a good purpose.

So is it okay to take your child there on Sunday night if you think he has strep throat? I would advise you to call your doctor first, but if you do go to a clinic, follow up with your pediatrician as soon as possible. If I couldn't get to my pediatrician's office, I'd feel relatively comfortable using one of these clinics for the following common problems:

- Swimmer's ear
- Rashes, poison ivy, bug bites, hives, or severe sunburn
- Pinkeye (conjunctivitis)
- Strep throat symptoms (requiring a culture test for strep throat)
- Splinter removals
- Cuts or bruises that don't require stitches

The American Academy of Pediatrics opposes the use of retail clinics for children and adolescents, though, because it feels pediatricians use even minor visits to address family issues and to check on immunizations, among other things. The AAP is also worried about continuity of care, which is a concern I share, too. In sum, use them if you're in a pinch, but let your doctor know so that he has a record of the illness and what was done about it.

Speed Bumps Happen

Sometimes, a relationship with a doctor can hit a speed bump— a conflict of opinions, a failure to communicate, a misunderstanding that gets tense. Now what? Here are some ways to ease through a potential rough patch with your pediatrician.

- If you disagree about something—say, the need to repeat a blood test on your kid several times to make triply sure a disease isn't missed—have a prompt conversation with the doctor (*without* your child present) and express your concerns. You both have your child's best interests at heart. Don't let things fester.
- If a medication or some other treatment is prescribed, ask your doctor how long it should take to work and what to do if it doesn't. And if you think it doesn't, call and calmly explain the facts. Ask if something else can be tried or if there is any other condition or disease that might have been overlooked. This is perfectly acceptable language as long as there's no accusatory tone. Talk through all possible courses of action. Maybe the problem is less medical and more behavioral and it's time to try a therapist. Doctors want to help, but try as we might, we're not perfect.
- Don't hesitate to bring up an iffy experience in the office, whether it was from the front desk, from the business administrator, or in the exam room. If you felt rushed, say so. If you need more information, speak up. We want to do the best job possible, but we're not clairvoyant. Feedback is great, and I welcome it.

Time to Fire Your Pediatrician?

If you have a pediatrician who would fail the vigorous "exam" outlined in this chapter or who just frustrates you (do you tend to leave the office more confused than when you entered?), you and your child deserve better. There are many things that could spur you to tell your pediatrician sayonara, but here are some of my deal breakers:

- It takes months to get an appointment.
- The wait time to be seen for a scheduled appointment regularly exceeds twenty to thirty minutes (and the parent and child are on time).
- The doctor didn't return an after-hours phone call or page within sixty minutes. (During busy office hours, give your doc a little more time.)
- The pediatrician was of little help during a hospitalization or an emergency situation.
- There's a pattern of the pediatrician not answering questions or dismissing multiple questions as unimportant.
- When the pediatrician was out, there wasn't adequate backup (referring patients to a hospital emergency department instead of having another doctor cover isn't adequate).

Resources for General Health Information About Children

American Academy of Family Physicians (AAFP) (www.family doctor.org)
Explore a wealth of practical information on diseases, conditions, medications, symptoms, healthy living, and more.

American Academy of Pediatrics (AAP) (www.aap.org)
Go straight to the Parenting Corner for advice on choosing a physician, immunizations, child development, safety and injury prevention, and more.

Centers for Disease Control and Prevention (www.cdc.gov)
This is the place for official government health data and recommendations for kids from birth to age twenty. You will find interactive tools, charts, growth tables, recommended vaccinations,

and information on infectious and chronic diseases, injuries, disabilities, and environmental health threats.

KidsHealth (www.kidshealth.org)
Here you'll find practical, easy-to-read articles on a range of diseases and chronic conditions. There are also doctor-approved resources and information. The site is divided into unique areas for parents, children, and teens.

U.S. Department of Health and Human Services (www.health finder.gov/kids/)
Check out this site with your kids! Includes games, contests, pointers on how to surf the Net safely and create personal sites, plus information on substance abuse, safety, and more.

Yuckiest Site on the Internet (www.yucky.com)
Explore a range of fascinatingly yucky science topics with your kids. The site includes a section on understanding the gross and cool human body.

CHAPTER 2 POP QUIZ ANSWERS

1. When shopping for a pediatrician, what should you always ask the pediatrician's office manager? The answer is D, all of the above. (Page 45.)

2. A parent who's tempted to call an ambulance every time her child skins a knee would probably be best served by a pediatrician whose treatment style . . . The answer is B. This parent should seek out a pediatrician who usually takes a more relaxed "watch and wait" approach. (Page 54.)

3. How long is too long to regularly wait in a pediatrician's waiting room? The answer is B, twenty to thirty minutes. On occasion you may get a longer wait, but with children in the equation, you need an office that keeps things moving. (Page 70.)

4. Even in a pinch, you should *not* use a retail health clinic (often found in pharmacies) to treat your child for . . . The answer is C, breathing difficulty. (Page 68.)

5. Never tell your child that a shot . . . The answer is B. Can you believe that a lot of parents actually use this threat? (Page 62.)

6. Which of these is something many pediatricians consider a time-wasting pet peeve? The answer is A. (Page 66.) You know, that doorknob thing!

7. What is *not* a legitimate reason to give your pediatrician the boot? The answer is B. On the contrary, refusing to give you an antibiotic even when you lay on the pressure is probably a sign that your doctor is quite prudent. (Page 69.)

Chapter 3

What's the Best Way to *Keep* Kids Healthy?

Nine Tips to Outwitting the Lure of Fast Food and Late-Night TV

POP QUIZ

Keeping children healthy—let alone happy—is a concern for all parents. Take this quiz to find out how much you know about keeping your child healthy. You'll find the answers to the questions at the end of the chapter. If your results are less than desirable, have no fear! After reading this chapter, you will know the answers to these questions and much more. Good luck!

1. Which of the following childhood illnesses has made a comeback in recent years due to unvaccinated children?
   A. Measles
   B. Rheumatic fever
   C. Polio
   D. Hoof-and-mouth disease

2. A study conducted by the American Heart Association found that the plaque buildup in the neck arteries of obese children or those with high cholesterol was similar to . . .
   A. Crisco
   B. The plaque buildup typically seen in forty-five-year-old adults
   C. The plaque buildup typically seen in seventy-year-old obese adults
   D. A golf ball stuck in a garden hose

3. What's a good way to determine the right food portion for a toddler?
    A. The portion should be about the amount of food he can stuff into his cheeks, like a squirrel.
    B. The portion should be one tablespoon of each food group (poultry/fish/lean meats, vegetables, fruits, whole grains) for each year of a toddler's age.
    C. Each portion should be about the size of the child's fist.
    D. Convert your child's body weight into grams, then divide by seven. The result is how many ounces of food your child should eat at each meal.

4. What should you never say to your child at mealtime?
    A. "Clean your plate."
    B. "When I was a child, there was no such thing as leftovers."
    C. "In Burma, people eat this all the time."
    D. "If you're not hungry, you don't have to eat your dinner."

5. How many hours of nightly sleep do experts believe most kids age seven to twelve need?
    A. Seven to eight
    B. Nine and a half
    C. Ten to eleven
    D. Twelve to thirteen

6. Between ages two and seventeen, what is the maximum amount of *total* "screen time" (TV, computer, video games, etc.) any child should have every week?
    A. As much as her agent can get her
    B. Twenty-two hours
    C. Fourteen hours
    D. One hour for every year of her age

As a parent of a baby, toddler, adolescent, or even early teen, you're probably looking forward to the day when this parenting thing gets easier. Me too! And it will get easier, but trust me, it will never be *easy*. We can't wave a magic wand and make our kids healthy, independent, and wise. Or thoughtful, appreciative, and punctual. Or neat, sweet, and with their pants worn at least somewhere near their waist. But we can point them in the right direction . . . and make sure that if they do screw up in a major way, it isn't because they imitated us. Here are nine tips that will help.

TIP 1: Help Your Child Be a Super Germ Fighter

Germs. They're about the only things that kids do voluntarily share, right?

No parents want their kids to be sick, but getting sick occasionally helps teach children's bodies to fend off infections. So the next time your child has a miserable cold or flu, try to remember that it's helping to build his young immune system. That's why it's perfectly okay—even beneficial—for youngsters to get sick a few times a year. In fact, the average child gets five to nine colds a year. (And you thought it was just your child.)

Young kids who catch fewer colds may pay the price later on. One study found that children who went to day-care centers (which are chock-full of germs because they're chock-full of kids) initially got sick more often than children who didn't go to day care—but they also had stronger immune systems by the time they started school. Children who didn't go to day care got sick more often during the first few years of elementary school. It would be interesting to follow up with these children in seventy years or so; I wonder who will have the last cough.

Some immunology experts believe that a baby's early exposure to germs may help him fight off allergies and asthma later in life. The jury is still out on that, but a small study has found that babies raised in homes with several pets have fewer allergies by age six or seven.

So Why Fight Germs?

As I said, germs are good in moderation. Some illness is inevitable, and usually it's not a big problem. Unfortunately, most germs don't understand the concept of moderation. They invade and attack our bodies as savagely as our immune systems allow.

Your mission, therefore, is to teach your child good, practical, lifelong habits that will let him avoid as many day-to-day germs as possible—both to avoid preventable illnesses that could become serious and to reduce the chance that he'll pick up a rogue bug (like MRSA; see page 11) that will outfox his immune system and make big trouble.

How Germs Spread

You can blame 80 percent of all infectious diseases on "contact spread." That includes direct person-to-person contact, such as touching or kissing, and indirect contact, such as when your child touches a contaminated table, toy, or doorknob and then touches his eyes, mouth, or nose. Since viruses and bacteria can live two hours or longer on cafeteria tables, keyboards, doorknobs, desks, and thousands of other surfaces . . . well, it's a jungle out there.

The most effective way to prevent contact spread is—you guessed it—frequent hand washing. Kids learn by example, so make sure you wash *your* hands frequently and thoroughly. **You need to lather up with soap and warm water for at least fifteen seconds to remove 90 percent of germs,** so teach your child to wash her hands for as long as it takes to sing "Happy Birthday" or the "ABC" song. (Of course, you may first need to teach her these songs.) This lesson can benefit your kids for a lifetime.

Waterless hand sanitizers are good when you're on the go. Keep them handy to use at the park or grocery store. Make sure your child rubs his hands until the gel is dry so the alcohol in it

Which Is Better: Antibacterial Soap or Plain Old Soap?

Cleansers with antibacterial chemicals are un-doubtedly effective. A study done in a class-room found a 50 percent drop in respiratory illness, a 35 percent decline in doctor's visits, and a 50 percent drop in absenteeism when antibacterial soaps were used and surfaces were cleaned regularly with disinfectants. However, in my home, I use regular soap, as there is some thought that antibacterial soaps may contribute to the development of stronger, drug-resistant bacteria in our environment, which is the last thing we need (see page 11). And if you're conscientious about washing, plain soap cleans hands nearly as well as antibacterial soaps.

kills the germs. Sanitizers don't do much for visible grime or grit, but they're better than nothing at all.

Germ Busters for Babies

- Don't worry if your baby pees in the bathtub. Believe it or not, urine is sterile!
- For the first six months of her life, limit the number of people who handle your newborn (and I don't just mean sketchy strangers). Ideally all would-be holders would do a thorough hand washing first. But I know this can be awkward. So carry a hand-sanitizing gel and ask people to use it before holding your baby. Just say it's doctor's orders. Because, well, it is.

- Check out your day-care center's policy about hand washing and diaper changing, and see what they do about potentially contagious children. Licensed day-care centers are required to have infection-control policies, so ask to see them.
- Clean dropped pacifiers with soap and water. Pet peeve alert: *Please* don't clean your baby's pacifier by licking it yourself. The human mouth has more bacteria than the mouths of many animals! Yuck. To get them really clean, throw those binkies in the top rack of the dishwasher. The covers that come with some pacifiers should also be washed regularly.
- Never spoon-feed your baby food straight from the jar and then return the half-empty jar to the fridge. Double-dipping can allow bacteria to grow in the food, which could make your

Put the Skids on Traveling Germs

Taking a trip with your children, especially overseas, means upping your vigilance. A child's immune system is still developing, so it's okay to be a bit fanatical about germs—especially in countries where hygiene standards might be less than perfect. Make regular and frequent stops to wash hands, especially in airports and at tourist attractions. Use only bottled water for drinking, tooth brushing, and mixing formula. Load up on alcohol-based hand sanitizers.

Pack prepackaged snacks for your children. While local fresh fruit may look healthy, I recommend eating only fruit with peels or rinds, such as bananas, oranges, and melons. Avoid other kinds of fruit, which might have been washed in iffy water or not at all.

baby sick after the next feeding. Spoon out a portion into a bowl, tightly cap the jar, and refrigerate it for later.

TIP 2: Help Your Child Stay at a Healthy Weight

Raising your child to eat nutritious foods and maintain a healthy weight is one of your most important jobs as a parent. Your child's eating and exercise habits will largely determine whether he'll enjoy a long, healthy life or a shorter one riddled with issues ranging from low self-esteem and depression to early diabetes, orthopedic problems, sleep apnea (episodes of interrupted breathing during sleep), and eventually heart disease, kidney and liver failure, and more.

Yes, this is all pretty scary stuff. But it's *all* preventable.

Know Your Child's BMI

How do you know if your child is overweight? Along with your pediatrician's judgment, a good indicator is your child's body mass index, or BMI. This number is based on your child's height and weight. If your child has a BMI higher than 95 percent of other kids in the same age, sex, and height group, that's considered obese. There are a number of websites that will automatically calculate your child's BMI if you punch in a little info. (Try this one: apps.nccd.cdc.gov/dnpabmi. Hint: Don't use an adult BMI calculator; the formula is different for children.) If doing math tickles you, however, you can figure out your child's BMI with these steps.

1. Measure your child's weight in pounds.
2. Measure your child's height in inches, and multiply that number by itself (if he's 58 inches tall, that would be 58 × 58, which equals 3,364).

3. Divide your child's weight by the figure you just calculated in step 2.
4. Multiply the resulting figure by 703.

For example, if your seven-year-old son weighs 80 pounds and is 4 feet 10 inches tall (58 inches), your calculation would look something like this:

$$58 \times 58 \text{ (or } 58^2 \text{ for you math whizzes)} = 3,364$$
$$80 \div 3,364 = .0238$$
$$.0238 \times 703 = 16.72$$
$$\text{BMI} = 16.72$$

By looking at the boys' BMI chart found at www.cdc.gov/growthcharts/, your son's BMI of 16.72 falls in the seventy-fifth percentile, which means he's a normal, healthy weight.

A Weighty Battle

There are a thousand important reasons to make sure your child adopts healthy eating habits and keeps a normal weight. However, it can seem like there are just as many factors that sabotage your efforts.

First of all, by the time your child is four or five, it's hard to control everything he eats. What goes on at home may be healthy, but what happens when he goes to a friend's house? Or eats at his school cafeteria? Or discovers fast-food chains? They sell happiness in a box: greasy, salty, fragrant food that comes complete with a plastic throwaway toy.

But there is good news: The government is getting tougher on advertisers and schools and encouraging restaurants to give children healthier options. Today, in many fast-food joints you can order apple slices instead of french fries and low-fat milk instead of a sugary soft drink. These choices didn't exist even a few years ago. In my home state, New York, fast-food chains have to list the calorie counts of foods on their menu boards. That's been a real eye-opener for many parents—and everybody else.

Naturally, however, almost all parents know that just *walking into* a fast-food restaurant and smelling those salty fries can destroy all hope of a healthy meal. You don't hear many kids screaming, "I want apple slices!" at McDonald's.

Another bit of cautiously optimistic news: Recent statistics suggest that child obesity rates have leveled off, after rapidly climbing for several decades. Give some credit to hard work by schools and parents, but don't celebrate yet. We still have *a lot* to do to get kids to eat smaller portions, devour fruits and vegetables, and be more active. None of these is an easy sell. But you will be doing your child a huge favor if you instill healthy eating habits early that will last a lifetime.

Old Before Their Time . . .

A study by the American Heart Association found that the plaque buildup in the neck arteries of obese children or kids with high cholesterol was similar to that of forty-five-year-old adults. The researchers concluded these kids—the average age was thirteen—should be treated as being at high risk for cardiovascular disease. Overweight teens can also suffer liver damage: Many obese teens might need liver transplants by the time they reach thirty, according to a study by the American Liver Foundation.

What Are *You* Eating?

Now for—*ahem*—your part: **If you want your child to eat a healthy diet, *you* have to eat a healthy diet.**

As parents, we're responsible for what our children eat—at least as long as we're in charge of their meals. And nothing has a more powerful influence on their eating habits than your eating habits. **If you don't eat healthfully, neither will your kids!** So make sure that you're a great role model. If you run around all day and only grab a candy bar and diet soda, or your usual dinner is a bucket of fried chicken wings, what kind of message does that send? Your kids are *always* watching you, so make sure you buy *and eat* food that's good for them and you. Then don't expect miracles. It might take a dozen attempts for your

Your Kid's Not Hungry? Doesn't Want Dinner? Don't Fret

When kids skip an occasional meal, it's usually no big deal. Elementary school children don't grow as quickly as adolescents do, so their energy needs remain lower until they reach puberty. (Then watch that grocery bill climb!) Even though you might feel sad because no one's eating your fine, home-cooked meal, try not to stress about a kid who would rather play than eat. In fact, as long as your child's growth is steady, encourage the playtime. That will fuel his metabolism and help him maintain a good body mass index (BMI). Just as long as high-fat, high-sugar, and high-calorie snacks, like cookies and chips, aren't replacing meals, skipping an occasional meal is fine.

child to give a healthy but "different" new food a try, but don't give up.

So, What Exactly Is a "Healthy Diet"?

When I say "diet," I'm talking about healthy, well-balanced eating, not about restricting calories. **Your child needs protein, carbohydrates, fat, minerals, vitamins, and fiber to grow and have energy.** And he should eat a wide variety of foods. Nothing should be off-limits. A healthy diet should be rich in fruits and vegetables but also include occasional treats so kids learn to enjoy them in moderation. How much food *your* child needs depends a lot on how active he is.

You're probably familiar with the best diet guideline—the government's Food Guide Pyramid. There's a pyramid online designed for kids age six to eleven that's been made into a computer game. Kids learn how to fuel a rocket with food and physical activity, then blast off. It's cute. Check out www.mypyramid.gov/KIDS. There's also a handy menu planner for moms and dads, and tips on getting kids to eat healthfully starting at a young age.

Toddlers: How Much Food Is Enough?

If your child is a toddler, serve portions that are right for his small size. Generally, a healthy portion is **one tablespoon of each food group for each year of your child's age.** Your two-year-old, for example, would get two tablespoons of each food group (poultry/fish/lean meats, vegetables, fruits, whole grains). It's fine to serve more if your toddler is still hungry.

Eight Rules for Raising Fit Kids

1. **Start feeding them healthfully** *now.* Even if your child is still a baby, begin keeping a wide selection of healthy foods at home. You want him to learn to eat nutritious food early—even if he doesn't have a clue what he's eating! The earlier he's exposed to good habits, the easier it will be to make them second nature.

2. **Limit fruit juice to six ounces a day.** Otherwise, he's filling up on juice and not drinking enough water and milk. Try to completely avoid sugary fruit punches and soda. They are full of sugar and empty calories and contribute to dental cavities and obesity in many children.

3. **Start the day with a hearty breakfast.** That goes for kids *and* adults. Try to include protein, whole grains, dairy, and fruit. Eating breakfast makes everyone less likely to overeat later in the day. Researchers say it's one reason people who maintain a normal body weight tend to be breakfast eaters.

4. **Never say "Clean your plate!"** This old parental guilt trip can backfire big time. Yes, children are still starving all over the world, but making your child overweight won't help them a lick. (I always wanted to say, "Please send them this," while sliding my plate of liver toward my mother.) So never badger your child to clean his plate. In fact, never force your children to eat. Offer healthy choices, and let your child decide how much to eat, within reason. Don't count calories either. Believe it or not, most kids know how much food their body needs at a sitting and self-regulate their eating.

5. **Don't use food as a reward.** Don't say, "You can play with your toys when you've finished all of your broccoli." You don't want kids to learn to eat when they're not hungry.

6. **Stock healthy snacks and make them appealing, fun, and easy to grab.** Think fresh strawberries, popcorn, crackers and cheese, crisp vegetables, low-fat yogurt, their favorite whole-grain cereals, and the like. Open your refrigerator

and cabinets, and stare. Brainstorm ways to make the healthier snacks more enticing to little eyes and hands, and easy to reach. Keep sliced fruits and veggies in the front of the refrigerator. Simply don't buy cookies, chips, and other junk food.

7. **Don't eat in front of the TV.** It's bad for everyone because it's so easy to zone out in front of the tube (or a computer screen) and mindlessly overeat. A recent study found that for every hour of TV watched, an average of 167 extra calories were consumed—mostly junk food.

8. **Don't let your child start drinking iced coffee or energy drinks.** In my opinion, that stuff is even worse than soda. It packs a wallop of sugar and caffeine but offers zero nutrition. Your child will crave more and more sugar and caffeine, which can have ugly side effects—poor sleep, mood swings, irritability, heart palpitations, jitteriness, and headaches. Caffeine-sensitive kids shouldn't have caffeinated sodas, tea, or even chocolate after lunchtime.

Follow the 10-2-0 Rule for Packaged Snacks

Check the label and make sure snack-sized packages contain no more than 10 grams of sugar, no more than 2 grams of fat, and 0 trans fat per package—not per serving. Don't be fooled by "snack packs" that have three or four servings rather than just one. Personally, I love the snack packs that have 100 calories each; they're a good way to keep treats under control, and it's easy to pair them with an apple or banana for kids on the go.

Preventing Eating Disorders

Eating disorders peak during puberty and the late teen/young adult years, but symptoms can occur earlier. The vast majority of sufferers are teen girls and young women, though preteens and boys can also get caught up in it. Denial is common in parents as well as kids, so don't convince yourself that your child is just "going through a phase." Seek professional help as soon as you notice any of the symptoms (see below). Delaying could make the road to recovery harder. Eating disorders are very serious but they're also treatable.

There are two main types that parents need to watch out for.

The first is **anorexia nervosa, a severe, life-threatening eating disorder.** What to watch out for: Sufferers are at least 15 percent below normal weight, are terrified of gaining an ounce, and obsess about their body shape and size. Other symptoms can include:

- Missed periods
- Fatigue
- Depression
- Lack of interest in school, friends, or activities
- Preoccupation with food (preparing it, counting calories, but not eating it)
- Secretive, self-induced vomiting (including use of syrup of ipecac)
- Laxative use
- Excessive exercising
- Anxiety at mealtimes
- Anemia
- Insomnia

One in ten people who battle anorexia die from severe weight loss, a weakened heart, or suicide. Survivors may suffer bone loss, infertility, and many other serious consequences.

The other major eating disorder is **bulimia nervosa. It's more common than anorexia but harder to detect because most sufferers aren't underweight.** Binge eating is followed by self-induced vomiting or other purging methods, often brought on by laxatives, diuretics, fasting, or excessive exercise, all used to avoid weight gain.

Millions of Americans suffer from binge eating, consuming eight thousand to ten thousand calories in a sitting. Fortunately, bulimia is rarely fatal, but it can cause tooth decay, hair loss, esophageal ruptures, and, in rare circumstances, cardiac arrest (especially when diuretic drugs or laxatives are involved). Left untreated, bulimia can lead to even more severe eating disorders. Symptoms can include:

It's a Thin-Obsessed World

 Some scary numbers from recent studies:

* 42 percent of girls in the first through third grades want to be thinner.
* 81 percent of ten-year-olds are afraid of being fat.
* 83 percent of sixth-grade girls diet occasionally.

Clearly, we have a lot of work to do in preventing eating disorders, starting with young children and with ourselves. Parents set the tone. Remember that what you do is much more powerful than what you say. The suggested tips on pages 84–85 can help you send positive messages to your child, but seek help immediately if you suspect your child has an eating disorder.

- Frequent bathroom trips after eating
- Evidence of binge eating, such as hoarded food
- Decayed teeth from vomiting
- A reddened finger from self-induced vomiting
- Unusually rounded cheeks (frequent vomiting can cause swollen glands)
- Lack of interest in school, friends, or activities
- Missed periods
- Preoccupation with food
- Laxative use

TIP 3: Make Sure Your Child Gets Enough Sleep

Is "Are you *still* awake?" an all-too-familiar refrain in your house? Is your kid's bedtime ritual a nightmare? For both of you? Boy, you are *so* not alone. I talk to parents all the time who are almost weepy about their youngsters' problems with sleep—or lack thereof. It affects everyone. Sleep troubles usually crop up at around five months and tend to improve after age four or so.

Some kids have trouble falling asleep or resist going to bed because they're afraid to be alone. Some have sleep terrors or nightmares, or snore loudly enough to wake themselves up (which could be a sign of sleep apnea and is worth discussing with your pediatrician). Some children crawl into their parents' bed in the middle of the night, swearing that it's the only place they can sleep (hey, kids can appreciate 350-thread-count sheets, too). Don't fall for it. Without creating a huge fuss, take your child back to his bed, reassure him, and tuck him in. If you give in to this habit, you will have a very hard time breaking it.

HOW MUCH SLEEP DO KIDS NEED?

Birth to 12 months old: 14 to 16 hours per day

1 to 3 years old: 12 to 14 hours per day

3 to 6 years old: 10 to 12 hours per day

7 to 12 years old: 10 to 11 hours per day

12 to 18 years old: 8 to 9 hours per day

Bedding Down by Age

Virtually all children have the ability to sleep well. They just need a little help.

Infants need routines but not strict schedules; begin to encourage babies three to four months old to fall asleep on their own. This is how they learn to soothe themselves.

Toddlers need routines that are consistently enforced; stuffed animals and blankies are encouraged, too. These transition objects allow children to feel safe and comforted when they are by themselves at night.

Preschoolers tend to develop creative stories and imaginations, so it's not surprising that this is when sleepwalking and night terrors tend to peak. Again, stick to a bedtime routine.

School-age children need regular, healthy sleep and *lots* of it. It's thought that most school-age kids age five to twelve actually get about nine and a half hours of sleep a night, but **sleep experts say that most need ten or eleven hours each night.** In battling the demands of after-school activities and sporting events, and then making time to eat and do homework, it's hard for a lot of kids to get to bed early so they're alert and well rested the next morning.

It *is* a juggling act, but you don't want your child to be sleep deprived from late-night homework (sometimes this happens, I know). Making it work may mean cutting out an activity or two, but you *can* make it work. See "Seven Ways to Be Sure Kids Get Their Zzzs."

Fast Facts: Kids and Sleep

❏ Kids who sleep fewer than nine hours a night are more likely to be overweight.

❏ During deep sleep, the blood supply to your child's muscles is increased, energy is restored, and tissue growth and repair occurs. All this means your child's body and brain are developing and growing, and his immune system is fighting sickness even while he sleeps. It's a beautiful thing.

❏ Children sleep fewer hours in the summer and on weekends.

❏ Kids (and adults, too) who use their bed just for sleeping (no laptop, no reading, no playing games, even no talking on the phone) sleep better because they've trained their body to associate their bed only with sleep.

❏ The National Sleep Foundation says that 26 percent of kids three and older drink at least one caffeinated beverage a day—and consequently lose thirty minutes of sleep nightly.

❏ Over-the-counter medications for cold and flu can keep your child awake. Ask your doctor before using these at night.

❏ Watching TV to wind down before bed might not work. The flickering electronic light from a TV or computer can stimulate the brain in ways that delay—by two hours—both the production of melatonin (the chemical the body makes to help us get sleepy) and the drop in core body temperature that makes us want to get under the covers. Yawn.

SEVEN WAYS TO BE SURE KIDS GET THEIR 222s

1. Set a regular time for bed each night, and stick to it.
2. Establish a relaxing bedtime routine for young kids, such as a warm bath and a story.
3. Make after dinner a slow-down time. Too much activity before bed can keep kids awake.
4. Avoid feeding children big meals close to bedtime.
5. Avoid giving children anything with caffeine (including hot chocolate and tea) within six hours of bedtime.
6. Make sure bedrooms are dark, cool, and quiet. Use a small nightlight only if necessary.
7. Keep computers and TVs out of kids' bedrooms—they encourage late-night "screen time" and you cannot monitor what they are viewing.

Adapted from the National Institutes of Health National Heart, Lung, and Blood Institute

❑ About 16 percent of kids snore, sometimes a few times a week. If you hear snoring or loud breathing from a kid, alert your pediatrician. Sleep apnea (episodes of interrupted breathing during sleep) is becoming more common in children, especially in those who are overweight.

❑ Sleep disorders can impair a child's IQ as much as lead exposure. Researchers have found that a child who snores and sleeps poorly will typically have behavior problems and an inability to concentrate.

TIP 4: Don't Fall Behind on Those Checkups

I know you *want* your child's eyes and teeth to stay as healthy as the rest of her body. Though many parents schedule regular checkups with their pediatrician, many do not. Nor do they schedule appointments for eye exams or teeth checkups. Don't fall behind or skip checkups! Some parents only take their children to a doctor when an illness or injury strikes. But when you skip a checkup, you're missing an opportunity to possibly catch or prevent a condition from developing. Regular vision and hearing screenings performed by your pediatrician or a specialist, like an ophthalmologist or ear, nose, and throat doc, and teeth checkups with your pediatrician (for babies) or dentist allow them to examine your child's body thoroughly and detect when problems—ones you might not notice otherwise—are developing.

Those Smiling Eyes . . .

First-time parents are surprised at how early babies need an eye exam. Newborns have their eyes checked before they leave the hospital; by the time they're six months old, your pediatrician will also have checked their eyes again for vision development and alignment.

Babies more than three months old should be able to follow a moving object with their eyes. If your child can't make steady eye contact or seems unable to see correctly, let your doctor know. It's normal for babies under four months old to occasionally cross their eyes. However, if it's happening a lot or you notice one eye turning in, tell your pediatrician. Your child's eyes should be checked by your pediatrician between ages three and four. Starting at age five, your pediatrician should check your child's vision every year.

If your child has an eye problem, or trouble reading or learning, your pediatrician may suggest seeing a pediatric ophthalmologist. These specialists can diagnose, treat, and manage all children's eye problems, including amblyopia or "lazy eye." Your pediatrician will likely suggest a specific doctor, but these two websites can also help you find pediatric ophthalmologists in your area:

- The American Association for Pediatric Ophthalmology and Strabismus (misaligned eyes): www.aapos.org (click on "Find a Pediatric Ophthalmologist")
- American Academy of Ophthalmology: www.aao.org/find _eyemd.cfm

And Those Smiling ... Teeth

Even though your little cutie will eventually lose all those sweet baby teeth, it's still important for kids to have oral health checkups. Your pediatrician can do this early on, but your child will need to start going to a dentist by age two or three (or sooner if there are signs of tooth decay).

From the time baby teeth arrive, it's important to clean them and the tongue twice a day using a soft washcloth or gauze with a small dab of nonfluoridated toothpaste. (I advise using nonfluoride toothpaste until at least age three, as swallowing too much fluoride can cause fluorosis—see page 276.)

From six months to twenty-four months, kids start teething in a major way, which makes them (and you) irritable. They'll bite on things, drool, and pull at their teeth. The simple, time-tested measures still work best: Offer a chilled teething ring or cold, wet washcloth. If you must use a pain reliever, I recommend Children's Tylenol (acetaminophen) or Motrin (ibuprofen).

By age nine, kids should be able to floss their own teeth, but you should start doing it for them before that, once they have

Some Dentists Prefer Pint-Sized Patients

If your regular dentist isn't great with kids, ask your pediatrician to recommend a pediatric dentist. Or check out the American Academy of Pediatric Dentistry website at www.aapd.org/finddentist/search.asp to find specialists in your area.

most of their baby teeth (or around age four). It's easier if you use fun prethreaded flossers meant for kids. By age seven or so, your child should be pretty expert at brushing—and the Tooth Fairy should make her first appearance. From ages six to twelve, it's normal for kids to have both baby teeth and some permanent teeth.

Don't forget to replace those bitten-up, worn-down toothbrushes every two to three months before they start breeding germs. That goes for your toothbrush, too!

TIP 5: Don't Miss Scheduled Vaccinations and Boosters

Unfortunately, 30 percent of kids in America aren't getting all the shots they need. That's more than scary, because missing even one shot could endanger your child's life and the lives of other children (and adults, for that matter). Unvaccinated children can spread disease to those who are too young or too medically fragile to be immunized. Also, there will always be some unvaccinated people among us—such as the elderly and people who lack health care—and having a high vaccination rate is the only way to protect them, by reducing the chance that they'll come in contact with an infected person.

Many American children who miss vaccinations have simply fallen through the cracks. They receive poor health care for a number of sad reasons, including a troubled family situation or outright neglect. But in a growing number of cases, the missed shots are no accident. Parents are *purposely* deciding to forgo vital vaccinations for their children. Why? Unfounded fears about vaccines are still spreading, including the baseless myth that autism is somehow linked to vaccines (especially the measles, mumps, and rubella vaccine, or "MMR" shot; see below for more on this). Misinformed parents are often scared by these rumors, and some react by leaving their children unvaccinated— making them vulnerable to deadly microbes that would just love a chance to kill or maim tens of thousands of people the way they did decades ago. These "cautious" parents don't remember the bad old days when children suffocated from diptherian membranes in their throat, fell into a coma from measles, were left sterile by the mumps, or died from meningitis.

Measles: Just a Plane Ride Away

As a direct result of these wrongheaded fears and rumors, there's anecdotal evidence that the rates of MMR vaccinations are declining—even though the law requires school-age children to receive MMR shots. (Exceptions are granted only to children with a history of severe reactions to vaccines or with fragile immune systems, such as kids with cancer.) If a rising number of children aren't getting this shot, we'll soon see the unmistakable sign: plenty of kids with measles spots. Measles is so contagious that it's often the first preventable disease to reappear when vaccination rates decline. And guess what? It's reappearing. More people in the U.S. had measles (131 cases) in the first seven months of 2008 than during any year since 1996, according to the Centers for Disease Control and Prevention (CDC).

The threat of measles is also only a plane ride away. While it

Pertussis Booster

Often thought of as a disease of ages past, pertussis—or whooping cough—is on the rise. To help prevent its spread, adolescents and parents of infants should get a booster vaccine, which is now combined with the adult tetanus/diphtheria vaccine. So, next time you need a tetanus booster (watch out for rusty nails), ask for the tetanus/diphtheria/pertussis combo booster. Your doc will be impressed!

may be rare in the U.S., the disease still rages in other countries. Not long ago, I received an alert from the American Academy of Pediatrics about a seven-year-old boy from San Diego who became infected with measles while in Switzerland with his family. He had never been vaccinated. When he got home, he gave the disease to his two siblings, five classmates, and four more kids who were at his doctor's office when he was there being diagnosed. None of these eleven children had been vaccinated either! It's easy to see how fast these things can spiral out of control (if you need a vivid primer, rent the Dustin Hoffman movie *Outbreak*). A measles epidemic anywhere in the world could make

In early 2009, Minnesota reported five cases of meningitis caused by Haemophilus influenzae type B (Hib), including an infant who died from the disease. Unfortunately, the infant had not completed the series of Hib vaccines, which have been available since 1992.

its way back to the U.S. within hours, thanks to plane travel. Foreign-born babysitters are also a known transmission source. (And Inga seemed so sweet.)

Bottom Line: Huge Benefits Outweigh Tiny Risks

When it comes to vaccinations, that's understating it. All my parents know my stance: It's *much* safer to receive all vaccinations on time than to risk a life-threatening disease. While no vaccine gives 100 percent immunity, we can largely thank vaccines for the robust health our children enjoy today compared to those of bygone eras. We now regard this good health as the norm. Many of us forget that a number of miserable diseases will return in a heartbeat if widespread vaccinations are ever interrupted.

Changing the Vaccine Schedule: Pros and Cons

Despite all the pleading and arm twisting by doctors and government health agencies, parents can choose not to vaccinate their children—if they're willing to risk the consequences. Some parents deviate from the vaccine schedule set by the CDC and the American Academy of Pediatrics because they feel it's better to space out the shots over a longer period of time. I don't agree, and there is no scientific evidence to justify spacing out the shots, but ultimately it's the parents' decision. However, they must understand the risks to their babies of delaying immunization.

> **FACT:** Vaccines save almost three million lives a year, according to the National Foundation for Infectious Diseases.

Some parents understandably want their infants to avoid the pain of several shots during one visit—but this means that they'll need more appointments. And if they don't stay on schedule, their children will fall behind on their immunizations and may never catch up. Still, a slow schedule is better than *no* schedule. So if parents are insistent about going slow, I will work with them as long as they fully understand the potential risks. But it is critical for them to adhere to the revised schedules. Besides the health dangers, public (and many private) schools will not accept children who are not vaccinated, with very rare exemptions.

If you have questions or concerns about vaccinations, have a talk with your pediatrician. This usually isn't a sixty-second conversation, so when you call the appointment desk, say that you want to talk about vaccinations and need time to discuss the issue. Boning up beforehand can help. Check these websites for more info:

- Johns Hopkins Bloomberg School of Public Health Institute for Vaccine Safety: www.vaccinesafety.edu
- The Centers for Disease Control: www.cdc.gov/vaccines
- American Academy of Pediatrics Immunization Initiative: www.cispimmunize.org

TIP 6: Monitor and Limit Your Child's "Screen Time"

Is your child, uh, electronically addicted? Glued to the TV, the computer, video games, or handheld electronic toys? Constantly texting friends on a cell phone? Most American kids over age five have at least one of these preoccupations, which their parents find grating (and gratingly expensive). But lest we forget, our generation spent endless hours playing Pac-Man and Super Mario Bros.—and our parents were certain it was turning our brains to mashed potatoes.

As much as we'd like to think so, we didn't have any more restraint back then than our kids have now; we just lacked today's technology. Our kids have access to digital TV with five hundred channels, an uncensored Internet with limitless content, and extremely realistic and violent video games that make our old friend Mario look like a kindly G-rated uncle. Which he was. His only fault was an intolerance of flying turtles.

Almost every parent can cite the dark sides of these new temptations. The Internet can allow dangerous strangers or even sexual predators to contact children. Kids can face daily or even hourly teasing, bullying, or harassment from their own school peers via e-mail, chat rooms, message forums, and text messages. Many teens and even preteens have engaged in "sexting," which can range from dirty talk on text messages to e-mailing nude photos of themselves. The list goes on . . . and we haven't even mentioned a subtler risk: All that sitting around while surfing the Net, watching TV, and sending text messages is helping to make our kids fatter.

A Sensible Solution: The Two-Hour Rule

Here's the number one rule to make sure that technology isn't a negative force: **Limit your child's total "screen time" to two hours a day.** Max. Including weekends. *Screen time* encompasses every possible activity that, well, involves a screen: using a computer, watching TV and DVDs, playing video games, text messaging, and otherwise gazing at any device that has a screen

FACT: Research shows that children who watch more than four hours of TV per day are more likely to be overweight than children who watch less TV.

attached to it (but don't count the time he spends standing at the porch's screen door staring outside).

To start, post a screen log where family members can keep track of their viewing time. You can copy the one below. Once you know how much time everyone spends watching TV and videos, playing games, and on the computer—and you recover from the shock—you can decide what steps to take next.

Screen Time Log

	TV (including DVDs, videos, etc.)	Video Games	Computer/ Internet	Cell Phone (texting, games, etc.)	Time (hours)
Monday					
Tuesday					
Wednesday					
Thursday					
Friday					
Saturday					
Sunday					
Total:					

Remember that the two-hour rule applies to children *over age two*. Children under two should have *zero* screen time, according to the American Academy of Pediatrics. And that means no *Baby Einstein* or other "helpful" DVDs marketed to parents of toddlers. A child's brain develops rapidly during the first two years of life, and TV and other distractions can get in the way of growing emotionally, socially, and physically. Babies need to play and explore, not sit and vegetate.

For children who are three or four years old, watching an hour

FACT: It's estimated that the average child will witness 200,000 violent acts on TV by the time he turns eighteen.

or two of high-quality educational programming each day—such as *Dora the Explorer, Blue's Clues,* and *Sesame Street*—is perfectly fine. Research has even shown that watching educational programs can improve reading and math skills in preschoolers.

However, please don't use this as an excuse to park your child in front of the TV for hours! Many parents do. It's understandable, especially during a stressful day. I've been there. The TV is so close, and you don't have to pay it $9 an hour to amuse your kids. However, *any* interaction your child has with another human being—reading together, playing a board game or ball game, dressing up dolls, anything—is almost always better for your child than watching TV.

If It's Turned On, They Can't Tune It Out

Don't use your TV as background noise. A study in the journal *Child Development* found that even if children aren't watching the TV, simply having it on in the room decreases the time they spend playing with toys—which fosters learning much better than passive activities (like staring at a screen). So when your child isn't watching a show, turn the TV off. Background music is a better option—though if it's heavy metal or hard-core rap, maybe not so much.

What Are *You* Watching?

You knew this was coming, didn't you? Your TV and technology habits set the same example for your child as your eating habits do. If you bury your head in a laptop for three hours every night or only know what day it is by the TV lineup, your kids will follow suit. Why shouldn't they?

TIP 7: Be Aware of the Stress in Your Child's Life

After age five or six, your child's sense of self-consciousness will develop, and she'll become aware of the many wonderful, terrible, grandiose, and petty things that exist in her small world. We might call it "Welcome to Life, Part II." The struggles, opportunities, and tribulations of normal childhood can create extremely stressful periods. Many kids will occasionally feel overwhelmed. Of course, extreme stress can strike earlier or more severely if your child's confronted with a big life issue: a divorce, the death of a parent or sibling, a serious illness, or countless other crises and calamities.

While some stress is necessary to teach children how to cope with ordeals, severe stress can weaken children's confidence and create a kind of static in their heads that they find hard to block out. Left unchecked, chronic childhood stress can lead to severe behavioral issues and evolve into a number of adult illnesses, including eating disorders, alcoholism, depression, and other serious diseases.

Nip It in the Bud

How can you help your child keep stress from getting to be a problem? When you sense that your child is upset about something, mention it and ask him to name the feeling. This will help him learn it's okay to talk about his feelings and that you're a source of support. (Hint: Even if he tells you something that makes you very angry, don't fly off the handle—it will transmit the exact opposite message.) Offer comfort, and help him come up with solutions for the stressors, whether it's a tough project at school, not fitting in with friends, getting cut at a sports tryout, or failing a test. Just don't try to helicopter in and solve all your child's problems yourself.

When you help build your child's tolerance for dealing with the ups and downs of life, you help him develop a stronger sense of self and the capacity to face an obstacle, deal with it, learn from it, and move on.

WHAT MAKES A CHILD RESILIENT?

- Feeling good about himself, having a healthy self-esteem, and knowing his strengths and weaknesses
- Having a sense of belonging, both at home and at school
- Being involved in the community through sports, art, drama, music, or religious groups
- Learning that it's okay to fail and try again but not to give up
- Understanding that temporary situations won't take over his life; learning to find the positive in negatives
- Developing empathy, understanding, and tolerance for others
- Learning how to set goals, organize, and work well with others

Today's Agenda: School, Soccer, Piano, Dinner, Cub Scouts, Homework, Science Project...

A national poll found that 80 percent of parents with kids age two to eleven said that parents today overschedule their children. Yet only one in eight thought *their* child was overscheduled. ("Overbook *my* child? *Moi?*") From the children and parents I see, I strongly suspect it's much more common than one in eight. Many children are *way* overbooked with activities, and it's their parents' doing. Some parents seem to think the more a child does, the better. Not true.

But I empathize. We all feel the pressure of wanting to be great parents and have talented, happy, and content kids, but are you stressed out from trying to raise a superchild? It's easy to get caught in this web, especially when your best friend tells you that her eight-year-old is excelling in gymnastics, French, molecular biology, and the cello. Parents experience peer pressure, too.

While it's important to expose your children to new ideas and experiences, you really want them to *persevere with an activity they are good at and find enjoyable.* That last point is key. When kids excel at something they enjoy, it makes them feel empowered to try other new activities.

Yet parents must also recognize the importance of downtime. Unscheduled free time allows kids to read a book, listen to music, ride a bike, play with a friend, and engage their imagination. Or take a nap!

Please, don't get me wrong. Structured activities are important and very positive experiences for children. But there needs to be balance in a child's life that includes downtime and family time. Personally, I allow my children two or three structured, preplanned activities a week. I'm teaching them how to manage their time so they can juggle schoolwork, sports, reading, chores, family activities, sleeping, and everything else. (I also *schedule* family meals, by the way, because it's so easy for them to disappear in the shuffle.)

How can you tell if your kids are overscheduled? Start by asking them, and yourself too. Then watch. Are they up until midnight doing homework? So wound up that they have trouble falling asleep? So tired that they're comatose at breakfast? Now, look at *your* schedule. Are all of the activities in your life, including your children's activities, impinging on family time? Are you often frazzled, running from one thing to the next? Are you overwhelmed or short fused by the end of the day because of all the running around?

Dealing with Peer Pressure, Teasing, and Bullies

Is your seven-year-old afraid to go to school or even to the playground? He's not alone. Bullying is epidemic, and hurtful teasing can start early, even in preschool. By the second grade, it can be prevalent. Bullies today come in all shapes and sizes. They don't necessarily look like the oversized cartoon bullies who like to threaten other kids. Even usually nice children can cave in to peer pressure and torment others about their weight, bad skin, "dorky" clothes, or nerdy glasses. Children also form cliques, and they can be cruel in excluding others. Being able to hide behind a screen on the Internet or cell phone emboldens many kids to harass others.

"You Gotta *Promise* Not to Do Anything"

Three-quarters of kids say that at some point they have been teased or bullied, verbally or physically. Yes, some of this is inescapable for all children, and in mild doses teasing can be a normal part of learning to deal with others. But when does it cross the line? If you notice that your child is anxious, preoccupied, not looking forward to school (school avoidance is a big tip-off), plagued by unexplained stomachaches or diarrhea, reticent about certain topics, or otherwise acting strangely, it's time to probe.

It may take some pushing from you because most kids *want to keep it a secret*. Often, they're ashamed or afraid to "tell" or scared that they'll make the tormenting worse if their mom calls the teacher and makes a fuss. (Most kids think, "At least now I'm getting teased only for being a weirdo and a wimp. If Mom and the teacher get involved, I'm a weirdo, wimp, rat, crybaby, and mama's boy.")

If you suspect your child is being bullied, ask questions like "What do you do at recess?" or "Who do you sit with at lunch?" (Actually, you should be asking these questions anyway. That way, you'll be more apt to notice if something is up.) Quietly talk to your child's teacher and ask if your kid is the butt of mean

I Suspect My Child Is a Bully . . . Now What?

If you think your child is guilty of picking on others, you need to have the "that is not acceptable" conversation. Ask your child if he's frustrated or angry about something. Is he a leader or a follower who is trying to fit in? Talk about alternatives to violent or intimidating behavior. Find out how you can help, but lay out consequences if the behavior doesn't stop. Ask his teacher, coach, or counselor for help. Many schools have good bullying prevention programs. Also, spend some time at stopbullyingnow.hrsa.gov. The site details initiatives in towns across America that are working to educate and engage students, parents, and their schools in bullying prevention.

jokes or tricks. You can help your child deal with cruel children by talking to him about it and, depending on your child's age and the severity of the situation, brainstorming solutions.

First, encourage your child to tell an adult if he's being bullied. Whether it's you, a teacher, a coach, or even a neighbor, an adult can help. If he's too afraid to tell an adult, encourage him to tell a trusted friend, brother, or sister who can offer help and support and who can approach an adult about the issue. Then give your child some tips to avoid these situations. For instance, staying in a group, joining clubs, or participating in activities where he can make friends are some ways to avoid bullies. Also, tell your child that if he feels safe, it is okay to stand up for himself by saying "Stop it!" and walking away.

TIP 8: Help Your Child (and You) Survive Puberty

The first thing you need to know is that puberty—that time when girls and boys develop secondary sex characteristics and fertility and start becoming young women and men—arrives on a different schedule for every child. At the same time, puberty is occurring earlier in general, so don't be alarmed if you notice changes at a younger age than you experienced. Typically, puberty in girls starts between eight and thirteen, and in boys between nine and fourteen. Yes, girls start earlier, which is why they're often uncomfortably taller than boys in junior high. Puberty can last a few years, so don't expect this ride to be short.

In girls, the first thing you will notice is small breast bud development, followed by pubic and armpit hair. About two and a half years later, they'll experience a growth spurt, usually followed by menstruation. The initial sign of puberty in boys is typically an increase in the size of the testicles and penis. Next pubic hair and armpit hair arrive, and then a deepening voice and increased muscle mass. Both girls and boys will experience some other pleasantries, such as acne and sweat gland development (read: body odor). All of these changes make for great consternation and chatter among kids. It's an incredibly awkward time.

Then, of course, there are the infamous roller-coaster emotions. Kids will be happy one moment and furious (usually at you) the next. Suddenly they'll want protection and coddling, and then independence and privacy. Naturally, they'll also begin to notice the opposite sex and get crushes, face peer pressure, and struggle with body image and self-esteem. It won't be easy. For anybody.

Early and Late Puberty

When puberty is well ahead of schedule—termed early puberty, premature puberty, or precocious puberty—it's usually not medically worrisome, but it needs to be checked out. Body fat can sometimes affect when puberty begins, so if your child is overweight, puberty may be earlier.

Premature puberty is more common in girls, who can start developing breasts and pubic hair before seven or eight. In boys, premature puberty can cause a deeper voice, growth spurts, and acne before nine. If your child may be experiencing early puberty, talk to your doctor about evaluation and testing. While it certainly doesn't mean there's a medical problem, it's a good idea to be sure.

The same holds true for late puberty. A doctor should make sure nothing is amiss. Girls are considered delayed if they don't develop breasts by age fifteen or haven't started menstruating by sixteen (or within five years of developing breasts). Boys are considered delayed if there is no testicle development by fourteen and if development of the male organs isn't complete within five years after the onset of puberty.

If your child is early or late, your doctor might run blood tests to check on hormone and thyroid levels or X-ray the wrist

Am I Normal?

Really, isn't that what we all want to be? (Well, most of us.) It's important to get comfortable talking to your child about puberty—what it means and what the physical and emotional changes will be like—before age eight. That may seem young, but some girls are already wearing training bras at that age. Start the dialogue little by little so it becomes "normal" to discuss these changes before and as they happen. Some schools teach kids about puberty, but others do not. Find out what your child may or may not be learning so that you can round out the information. Also, not all of your child's playground "sources" will be reliable. So consider . . .

* telling your child when you learned about puberty and how the changes made you feel
* talking about one positive and one embarrassing experience you had during puberty
* relaying what you wish someone had told you beforehand
* sharing photos of yourself before, during, and after puberty
* buying a child-friendly book (or two) about puberty and body changes that answers questions your kid may be too embarrassed to ask and that never crossed your mind

to see if bone growth is normal. If those tests don't turn up any clues, your doctor may suggest further testing, which may include chromosome testing or possibly a CT or MRI scan of the head to rule out a tumor. Other imaging testing may be needed to evaluate the ovaries and testes. If your child has late puberty, your doctor may suggest seeing a pediatric endocrinologist who specializes in growth and hormonal disorders for further evalu-

MY DAUGHTER IS TWELVE AND WANTS TO USE TAMPONS; IS THIS OKAY?

A female who is menstruating can use a tampon at any age. Many of my young female patients, especially those who participate in activities such as dancing, gymnastics, running, and swimming, use tampons.

The only requirement is that a young woman be mature enough to use them responsibly. She must understand that tampons must be changed at least every six hours to avoid health risks (such as toxic shock syndrome, or TSS, a bacterial infection that can occur if a tampon is left in for too many hours). She also needs to understand the necessity of good hygiene, such as washing her hands before and after removing a tampon.

Some young women may find inserting the tampon tricky or slightly uncomfortable due to the hymen—the small membrane over part of the vaginal opening that is intact in sexually inactive females. Slender tampons with a plastic applicator that has a rounded tip may be easier to use. Smaller, thinner tampons made just for teens may be more comfortable but need to be changed more frequently. Teens should use the least-absorbent tampon they can based on their flow each day, which will also help prevent TSS.

ation. But most of the time, no cause is found and no treatment is needed.

Finally, some kids with early or late puberty are the butt of teasing in school. If you suspect that's happening, see the section on bullying, page 105.

TIP 9: Don't Blink.

If you do, your child will be grown up. No study has proven this, but many very dependable sources have warned me that it's true. They say it's an incontrovertible fact and have urged me to take their advice. Take pictures. Take trips. Take problems in stride. Do not blink. Enjoy the youth and health of your children. One is momentary and the other is largely thanks to you.

I'm hoping they're wrong about this "in a blink" thing, but they sure sound convinced of it.

CHAPTER 3 POP QUIZ ANSWERS

1. Which of the following childhood illnesses has made a comeback in recent years due to unvaccinated children? The answer is A, with all of its miserable spots. (Page 95.)

2. A study conducted by the American Heart Association found that the plaque buildup in the neck arteries of obese children or those with high cholesterol was similar to . . . The answer is B—they're like a forty-five-year-old's. (Page 81.)

3. What's a good way to determine the right food portion for a toddler? The answer is B. Go find your measuring spoons! (Page 83.)

4. What should you never say to your child at mealtime? The answer is A, which should finally shut down the Clean Plate Club. (Page 84.)

5. How many hours of nightly sleep do experts believe most kids age seven to twelve need? The answer is C, but they only get an average of nine and a half hours, so they get about three hours less than they need. (Page 89.)

6. Between ages two and seventeen, what is the maximum amount of *total* "screen time" any child should have every week? The answer is C. They should get no more than two hours a day, or fourteen hours a week—and that includes doing homework on the computer and looking at anything else that has a screen: cell phones, TVs, video games, etc. (Page 99.)

Chapter 4

How Do You Cope with Asthma, ADHD, Autism, and Other Special Needs?

Finding Support and Managing the Diagnosis, the Records ... and the Stress

POP QUIZ

Raising a great kid may be the most rewarding thing you'll ever do, but—if you're a newbie, trust me—it will also be the most challenging. Ask any experienced parent! Now try raising a child who has special needs or a chronic illness. The challenges go off the charts. But the rewards can, too. Still, you need a lot more know-how under your belt. If you don't have a kid with special issues or you get a gold star on this miniquiz, feel free to skip this chapter. If not, it's a must-read. (As always, answers are at the end of the chapter.)

1. How many U.S. children between the ages of two and eighteen are estimated to have a chronic health problem?
   A. 7 percent
   B. 22 percent
   C. 30 percent
   D. 40 percent

2. What does "CSHCN" stand for?
   A. Children with Social Hygiene Concerns.Net
   B. Children with Special Health Care Needs
   C. Center for Special Hospitalized Children in Need
   D. Center for Shih Tzu Housing, Care, and Nurturing

3. Which of these statements about asthma is true?
   A. It can be cured if treated neonatally with common, inexpensive medications.
   B. In 50 percent of asthmatic children, it becomes inactive during the teenage years.
   C. Recent research has shown that it's largely a psychological condition.
   D. About 10 percent of asthmatic children will never have an actual asthma attack.

4. Which of these statements about attention deficit/hyperactivity disorder (ADHD) is true?
   A. About 80 percent of children grow out of ADHD.
   B. Recent research has confirmed that excessive TV watching and video game playing cause ADHD.
   C. About 50 percent of children who need medication for ADHD will still need to take medication as adults.
   D. About 9 percent of children with ADHD will end up in reform school unless they are treated.

5. Which of these historical figures is thought to have had ADHD?
   A. Julius Caesar
   B. Galileo
   C. Franklin Delano Roosevelt
   D. Howdy Doody ·

Get this: It is now estimated that up to 30 percent of children between the ages of two and eighteen in the U.S. have a chronic illness or condition. That number has more than doubled over the past twenty years. Put another way: Every day, more and more parents are confronted with the staggering news that their children will require special, long-term care. Maybe for months or years. Maybe forever.

Chronic health problems include asthma and serious allergies, which are by far the most common, but there are many others: cancer; Down syndrome; mental retardation and other types of developmental disorders, such as autism; diabetes; ADHD (attention deficit/hyperactivity disorder); epilepsy; cerebral palsy; hemophilia; and sickle cell disease.

Why are some of the numbers increasing so much? That's the $64 billion question. For certain conditions, such as autism, we don't know why cases are increasing so rapidly. Some researchers believe we can thank (or blame, depending on your viewpoint) better diagnostic tools, which means doctors simply are finding more cases, not that there necessarily are more. But others believe there must be environmental triggers that we're overlooking. Some conditions have fairly obvious causes—the spike in diabetes is almost certainly due to the rise in childhood obesity. But regardless of whether the causes are mysterious or blatant, the result is the same: More and more kids are in big-time chronic health trouble. And their parents are reeling.

All Different, All "CSHCN"

So what's a "chronic illness"? The general definition is any health problem that lasts more than three months and significantly affects a child and his family. Children who have chronic medical, developmental, behavioral, or emotional conditions are collectively defined as "children with special health care needs" ("CSHCN" for short, which makes for easier writing but doesn't do much for talking). This widely adopted term is now used to identify *all* kids who need extra health care, regardless of their condition.

Yes, I know, this definition seems absurdly broad. A child

with severe cerebral palsy who needs constant care and a child with moderate asthma who needs to keep an inhaler handy are both considered CSHCN. What could they possibly have in common? I mean, besides a love of SpongeBob Squarepants and cheese pizza? Not much. But their parents share several identical goals.

For starters, both sets of parents need to develop a solid, long-term plan for their child's medical care. Both must work hard to avoid—or minimize—known dangers and setbacks. Both need to view their child's condition as always there, even when everything is going well on the surface. Finally, both will face a labyrinth of health care decisions that can be almost impossible to navigate without hard-won insider knowledge. See pages 119–22 for myths and facts about five common chronic conditions.

Dealing with the Diagnosis

Hearing that your child has a chronic illness or special needs can be difficult, to put it mildly. For many parents, it's life changing. When my husband and I learned that our first child, Noah, had autism, it was an emotional time. I was already pregnant with my second child and we were both pressingly busy. Yet we knew we had to quickly learn an enormous amount in order to make wise decisions and get him the best care possible.

Parents who get this kind of news often go through the classic stages—denial, depression, guilt, and anger. Your child's diagnosis can leave you shocked and overwhelmed. You may feel lost and not know where to turn. At the same time, oddly, you may also feel relieved. If you've spent months trying to find out what's wrong with your child, getting an accurate diagnosis with an actual, concrete name can make you go, *"Finally."* At least you know what you're dealing with even if you don't yet know how you're going to deal with it.

All of these feelings are normal. Talking to other parents in a similar situation can help immensely. Your doctor, hospital, or school may be able to help you meet other families who are dealing with a chronic illness. You can check online websites for children and their families who are struggling with the same illness you are. (See a list of resources on page 151.) Local networking can lead you to support groups that can help your child, your other kids, and you cope better.

Many parents will tell you that it's essential to take things one day at a time—to stay focused on the present rather than melting down about the future. It will also help your mental state if you begin to tackle your first mission: getting the equivalent of a PhD in your child's condition. Immerse yourself in information from responsible sources. Your growing knowledge will make you feel empowered, and that will help you regain a small but precious sense of control. You'll feel proactive, and you'll be able to spot potential issues.

Your first information sources should be your pediatrician and the specialist who made the definitive diagnosis (if there was one). Lean on both of them. Ask them for books, pamphlets, or videos that will help bring you up to speed on your child's condition, and don't be discouraged if you need a wheelbarrow to transport everything to your car. Ask them as many questions as you can think of, and **buy a notebook** in which you can write down concerns and track medical appointments, people, tests, results, and treatments your child may need. Ask them to recommend good websites for basic information, support groups, blogs by parents in your situation, and other helpful resources. At the very least, knowing you are not alone is comforting and will give you strength.

Answers: On the Way?

It's unclear why so many more children today are suffering from diseases such as autism and ADHD, which were virtually unheard of a generation ago. We also can't fully explain why premature births, asthma, obesity, and several childhood cancers are skyrocketing. But kids today are surrounded by unprecedented levels of synthetic chemicals and toxins, whose long-term effects simply aren't known—and many pediatricians and researchers believe these elements somehow play a role in soaring childhood diseases.

Soon, however, we should start getting some insights. A comprehensive, twenty-five-year research project called the **National Children's Study** was recently launched by the National Institutes of Health and other federal agencies. It will closely monitor more than a hundred thousand children from before birth until age twenty-one to assess many of the possible effects of many things—from environmental pollutants to eating habits—on children's health. This study is one of the most exciting developments in pediatrics in decades, and the great hope is that it will yield clear-cut results and recommendations akin to those from the landmark Framingham Heart Study, which confirmed that high cholesterol, high blood pressure, obesity, and inactivity were indeed strong risk factors for heart disease. Stay tuned!

REALITY CHECK!
Myths and Facts About the
Five Most Common Childhood Disorders Today:
Autism, ADHD, Asthma, Diabetes, and Down Syndrome

Three Myths and Three Facts About Autism

Myth #1: A child with autism spectrum disorder (ASD) is unable to feel emotions or develop personal attachments.

Fact: Parents and family of a child with ASD need to learn how to show affection on the child's terms. The child may not be able to express his feelings well, but he does feel them . . . so much so that many people with ASD get married and have families.

Myth #2: All people with ASD have savant or special skills like Dustin Hoffman's character in *Rain Man.*

Fact: Only about 10 percent of people with ASD have special skills, and they usually appear in only one area; for example, your child may remember the birthday of every child in his class but may not remember their names.

Myth #3: Children with ASD cannot make eye contact or show affection.

Fact: Some children do make eye contact, and some work for years to learn to make eye contact. Showing affection is difficult for children with ASD, but it can be achieved if you model that behavior, be patient, and give it time. A child with ASD may be very affectionate, but he may not express it in traditional hugs and kisses.

Three Myths and Three Facts about ADHD

Myth #1: Poor parenting is to blame for ADHD behaviors in children.

Fact: ADHD is a physical disorder caused by differences in the way a child's brain works. Family conflicts or disruptions may aggravate ADHD but they don't cause it.

Myth #2: Children typically outgrow the symptoms of ADHD.

Fact: Sometimes the symptoms decrease during the teen years, but plenty of high school kids with ADHD find it hard to organize homework assignments and complete complicated projects. Some children have fewer symptoms as they reach adulthood, while others don't.

Myth #3: Children treated with ADHD stimulant medications can become addicted to them or become prone to drug abuse as they get older.

Fact: ADHD medications are not addictive when used as prescribed. In fact, treating ADHD with effective meds may actually reduce the risk of substance abuse.

Three Myths and Three Facts About Asthma

Myth #1: You cannot outgrow asthma.

Fact: In about 50 percent of children, asthma becomes inactive in the teenage years. The symptoms can recur at any time in adulthood, but they may not.

Myth #2: Asthma is a disease triggered by emotions.

Fact: Emotions don't cause asthma, even though emotional stresses—crying, yelling, or even laughing hard—can trigger symptoms. Asthma is a chronic disease in the airways of your child's lungs. It's always there, even when there are not a lot of symptoms.

Myth #3: A child with asthma can never play sports.

Fact: Many star athletes have asthma, including former Pittsburgh Steeler Jerome "the Bus" Bettis and Alberto Salazar, winner of the New York and Chicago marathons. (For more examples, see page 292.) Many take medication and work with their doctors to help prevent attacks.

Three Myths and Three Facts About Type 1 Diabetes

Myth #1: The reason some children get type 1 diabetes is because there's too much sugar in their diet.

Fact: Type 1 diabetes is caused by an autoimmune attack on the pancreas that destroys insulin-producing cells in the body. "Getting it" has nothing to do with eating too much sugar.

Myth #2: Children who do get type 1 diabetes should stop eating anything with sugar.

Fact: Kids with type 1 diabetes can eat sugar as long as it's counted as a carbohydrate and the proper amount of insulin is given to cover it. Keep an eye on fat and cholesterol intake, too.

Myth #3: Children with type 1 diabetes can't play sports.

Fact: Sure they can, as long as they check their blood sugar before playing and stabilize it if needed. It's also smart to have a source of sugar on hand, in case their blood sugar drops. Many successful athletes have diabetes, including baseball star Ron Santo, world-class surfer Scott Dunton, and tennis ace Billie Jean King.

Three Myths and Three Facts About Down Syndrome

Myth #1: Children with Down syndrome must go to segregated special schools and adults with Down syndrome usually must live in institutions.

Fact: Many people who have Down syndrome live with their families, are educated in mainstream classrooms, and hold various jobs as adults.

Myth #2: People with Down syndrome are severely retarded.

Fact: Most people with Down have IQs in the mid to moderate range of retardation, but Down kids can be educated and researchers are still discovering the full potential of people with Down syndrome.

Myth #3: Most Down kids are born to older parents.

Fact: While the incidence of Down syndrome does increase with the age of the mother, about 80 percent of children with Down syndrome are born to women younger than thirty-five.

Explaining an Illness to Your Child

If your child is diagnosed with a chronic condition as a baby (or even before birth), you may have years to prepare for telling her about the condition. But if your child is older, that conversation needs to happen much sooner—maybe pronto. And if the mere thought of that gives you night sweats, you're not alone. Many parents have a tough time deciding exactly how much or how little to tell their child.

From my experience, and that of social workers I've talked to, I believe that it's usually best to be candid with your child. Children are more perceptive than you might think. You don't want to cause unnecessary anxiety or stress, but you don't want to be dishonest either. If you mislead her, your child may feel confused or, worse, not trust you later. Ask your pediatrician for suggestions on how to explain a particular illness to your child.

My general advice—which, of course, depends on your child's age and maturity level and the specific condition you're dealing with—is to give your child the facts, but don't overwhelm her with details. Using simple terms that your child is capable of understanding, you may have to tell her that she's sick and will have to take medicine to breathe better. Or that she must now strictly watch what she eats and take daily medication to avoid becoming seriously ill from something called diabetes. Whatever the diagnosis, make sure your child knows *the illness is not her fault.* (Even if it *is* partially, due to persistent overeating or picking up a tick in the grassy lot where you forbade playing. Right now is not the time for an I-told-you-so speech.) A lot of young kids think an illness is punishment for something they've done, so you need to dispel that thought as quickly as possible.

Crying Is Good—in Private

To keep the lines of communication open, you're going to need to support your child, listen to her, and discuss her feelings about the illness. This will be hard, but save your tears for alone time because your child needs to feel that she can talk to you about the illness without *your* becoming upset.

Rather than making this talk a one-way medical lecture, ask how your child is feeling and listen to everything before offering explanations or more information. For many questions, you won't have good answers. Neither will your pediatrician. If your child asks, "Why me?" it's okay to say, "I don't know." If your child says, "It's not fair," agree. If your child is angry about the illness, let her talk about that until she gets her feelings out. If your child asks what caused the illness or condition, and the answer isn't clear, say, "I don't know," and stress the positive aspects of treatment and the prospect of improvement, if that's the case.

Again, above all, be honest. If there's a particularly difficult piece of information you're not sure it's wise to share, but your child is grilling you, ask your pediatrician for some guidance. It may be tempting to spring for a new bike, the latest video game system, or some other big treat to gloss over this difficult time, but that might be an iffy move. If there are many challenges to come, you'll need to devise ongoing helpful strategies that don't involve a constant stream of new stuff. Plus that can cause resentment among her siblings.

In the days, weeks, and months after "the talk" (it can make that birds-and-bees chat seem ho-hum), your child may have some rough periods. Just like adults, kids need time to adjust to the prospect of being sick. Your child may feel sad, depressed, angry, afraid—or deny that anything's wrong. Some kids don't want to talk to their parents about their concerns. That's fine. Just keep an eye and ear open, and be ready for a chat when they do. Children who have chronic illnesses often feel alone, different,

Your Child Is Listening . . .

 Be very careful about how you talk about a chronic condition if your child might be in earshot, or even in the same county. Kids have a way of walking into a room very quietly and overhearing phone conversations with doctors, calls with insurance representatives, or a heart-rending chat with your best friend where you let your fears flow. If you need to unload with another adult—and you will—do it when there's absolutely no chance your child will hear it.

and isolated—exactly the opposite of how most kids (and adults) want to feel. They just want to be kids and to be like their friends. Being around other kids with a similar condition can help a lot. That's another way hooking up with support groups can make a huge difference. Your child will benefit from knowing he's not alone, and he'll see how other kids are coping.

Finally, remember that kids' thoughts and feelings about their illness change over time. You may want to gently remind your child that the two of you can talk *any*time, now or in the future. If your child continues to be withdrawn or depressed, or isn't eating or sleeping well, much less talking, check with your pediatrician about getting professional counseling.

Remember the "Telephone" Game?

If your child is over age seven or eight, he'll likely ask you how to explain his illness to others. Work out a simple explanation together that he's comfortable with and can deliver, and offer to role-play with him what others might ask and how he might respond. If your child fears being teased, suggest some ways to handle that, too, such as ignoring comments or walking away. (See more about dealing with bullies on page 136.) Bottom line: Come up with a clear, simple explanation that your child completely understands and can field questions about. Otherwise, his version of "the talk" can turn into an error-laden mess when he tells his best friends and they tell his not-so-best-friends. So keep the message straightforward, short, and, if at all possible, upbeat.

Using Role Models

Celebrities have an amazing influence on society, don't they? For better and worse. Just switch on the TV or walk past the supermarket tabloids if you need a reminder of this. Perhaps you've already had your arm twisted to shell out for a pair of jeans, sunglasses, or a T-shirt endorsed by some boy-band singer who will be struggling to get on a reality TV show three years from now.

However, our celebrity-obsessed culture can sometimes be a real boon. Quite a few stars help with awareness about certain diseases. And a celebrity's influence can be especially strong medicine for a child coping with a chronic illness. Learning that a famous baseball player or pop star shares the same condition can be inspiring for a kid. (Of course, it can result in a whole new rash of merchandise and clothing requests, but those are the breaks.)

Do a little online research and see what famous or highly accomplished people your child might identify with, then use them to inspire and help him. For instance, did you know the famous Italian scientist, Galileo, was believed to have had ADHD? See appendix A at the back of the book for a quick sampling (and matching game) to get started.

Searching for Positives

Although there are many negatives about chronic conditions, there is a surprising number of positives, too. In studies of children with cancer, for instance, siblings said they felt closer to family members and developed increased empathy for others and respect for their ill sister or brother. Similarly, studies of kids with a developmentally disabled sibling found that they had better social skills ("an empathetic and caring nature"), likely because they understood the difficulties their sibling faced. Another study found siblings of children with diabetes were kinder toward others. So if your child's beefy older brother has recently stopped giving nerds swirlies in the elementary school bathroom, a whole crop of kids may owe your younger son's condition a debt of gratitude.

In real life, many of the parents I see who care for kids with special needs have noticed positive changes in their home life. I have, too. A parent of one of my special-needs patients calls it "the hidden silver lining." When one person is ill, the whole family often becomes closer. Some family members say they have matured in new ways and developed a more positive and humorous outlook on life, and more compassion and tolerance for others—traits that are truly needed in the world, I would say.

It shouldn't come as a surprise, however, that *you* chiefly decide whether you'll reap benefits from this difficult journey. As hard as it may be, try to view your child's illness as a challenge rather than as a daily threat or a loss. That will help you live with hope rather than fear or depression.

Preparing for Tests and Procedures

Unless your child is very young, you'll need to prepare him for whatever ongoing tests and medical procedures his condition requires. Kids need to know what to expect; worrying about unknowns can be worse than the real thing, so it's usually much wiser to be forthcoming. Lies can scar for life. Horror author Stephen King has written about an episode that illustrates this. When he was a child, a doctor put an instrument in his ear and told him he wouldn't feel any pain. Then the doctor lanced his infected eardrum to drain it—which ranks among the most painful procedures known to humankind. King never trusted doctors again, and I don't blame him. It might be the scariest thing he's ever written, and that's saying something.

If you're not comfortable preparing your child for a procedure—or you're simply not 100 percent clear yourself about the steps—there are a couple of things you can do. If you're in a hospital that has any "child life specialists" on staff, ask for one. Part of their job is to explain procedures and help kids deal with the anxieties that come along with being ill. (See more about child life specialists on page 212.) Otherwise, before the procedure starts ask whatever medical staffers are involved (doctors, nurses, technicians) to help you explain to your child what will happen and why it's necessary. What your child wants to know will chiefly involve these ten concerns:

1. What is being done?
2. How much will it hurt?
3. Why must it be done?
4. How much will it hurt?
5. Who will do it?
6. How much will it hurt?
7. How will these people do it?
8. How much will it hurt?
9. What equipment will be used?
10. Will any pain be involved?

Never-Ending Needles?

Some children with chronic illnesses or conditions learn one unpleasant fact rather quickly: Ongoing tests or treatments might mean getting pricked more than a pincushion. While no child (or adult) likes getting an injection, having blood drawn, or getting an IV inserted, children who frequently have to deal with needles may need extra coping help. First, ask the nurse or doctor to apply numbing EMLA cream to the injection site about one hour before the needle stick. Other tips:

- Explain the need for the needle in language your child will understand. You might say, "The doctors need to look at your blood so they'll know what medicines will work best," or "This shot will make you feel better."
- Don't fib and say the needle won't hurt. Tell your child it will pinch or sting for just a second or two and then go away.

- Distract your child with an iPod, stories, video games, or a coloring book so he's not obsessing over the needle stick.
- If your youngster needs regular shots, make a reward chart and offer a sticker or other small treat every time your child cooperates.
- If he's old enough, help your child feel that he can control some aspect of his situation, such as deciding which arm to have blood drawn from, or which day a test will be performed, or what treat he'll get for behaving well.
- If your child needs regular shots and his anxiety level isn't diminishing, find a different staffer or doctor to administer the shots, or ask if there's a child life specialist or social worker who can help ease his nerves. Don't stick it to your child by staying stuck.

Remember that the buildup before a shot is often much worse than the actual injection. I've had parents ask me to wait until their child is "ready" for a shot. If I actually waited until my patients were ready for shots, I'd be waiting forever. Children are never *ready* for a shot. My advice: Keep the pre-shot discussion brief, hold the child, and get it over with. Your kid will thank you in the end, and so will I!

Talking with Siblings

If you have more than one child, you know how different siblings are—and how easily they can become jealous if anyone thinks the parents are playing favorites. It's super-easy to get wrapped up in the well-being of the child with health problems and not notice fear, jealousy, anger, or loneliness brewing in your other kids. You will need to explain to them that a chronic illness is something their brother or sister may have for a long time, maybe always. Some conditions may improve over time (asthma); some can be managed by diet, exercise, and medication (diabetes); and some may go into remission (cancer).

Your other children may go through some profound changes and struggles as they try to grapple with what this means for their sibling, themselves, and the family. If the child who is sick needs special devices or medicines, your other children may be embarrassed by their sibling's condition—which is natural—but it's important to teach them about the condition and tell them that it is not a reflection on themselves. Other children may tease or be nasty because they don't understand the condition. When this happens, siblings can help allay fears and misinformation about their sib's condition.

Some illnesses mean a child will tire easily, need special foods, not play sports, miss a lot of school, use a wheelchair, or carry oxygen. Your child may look fine and function normally around others but require special care that his siblings need to know about. Be open about the condition, and make sure your other kids know that they can't "catch" the illness.

Young children sometimes think that their resentful thoughts ("I hate my brother; I wish he'd die") can actually cause illness or make it worse. Help your other kids express their feelings, and reassure them they are not to blame. Tell them they can help their sibling out with chores if your ill child isn't feeling well enough to contribute or by being quiet when he needs extra rest. If your child has asthma, his siblings can help him remember his inhaler for school or pick up homework assignments if he's sick or in the hospital. **But be careful not to put too much adult responsibility on your other children.** You don't want to take time away from their growing-up experience. The goal is to make sure no one in the family feels like they're losing out, or losing you, because of your special-needs child. Make sure you spend time together as a family, and also carve out special time for each sibling. You may want to set aside a night a week for each child (and a night for yourself and your partner!) to spend one-on-one time together.

Eventually, by the way, your other children will want to

know more about what's going on and perhaps get involved. If a sibling wants to come along on a hospital or treatment visit, that's lovely as long as the child is mature enough to handle it. Being together may add comfort during the treatment and understanding later on.

Being Ready for a Special-Needs Emergency

All parents need to be prepared for health emergencies (see chapter 5), but if your child has special needs, being prepared takes on a whole new meaning.

Kids with physical, cognitive, emotional, or social limitations are much more at risk for injury—which means they're more likely to end up in the emergency department than other kids. They may also be in more danger when they get to the ED. Children with special needs often have underlying problems that may be undetectable by an emergency physician who's treating the child for the first time. For instance, some children with chronic medical conditions have complicated drug regimes that can interact dangerously with common medications given during typical emergencies. (Check with your doctor or pharmacist to find out if your child is taking one of these meds.) Finally, it's very hard for emergency department doctors and nurses to be aware of every new treatment guideline for every disease. That's why you need to make sure that your child has a medical alert bracelet or other device. And that's why you always need to have a form handy that clearly spells out all of his key medical information. This form should include:

- all medications your child is taking
- any special emergency treatment restrictions your child's condition dictates
- any new or experimental therapy he may be receiving

Where can you find such a form? Just turn to page 133 for the one the American Academy of Pediatrics recommends. Fill it out, make multiple copies, and distribute it. Put a couple of copies in a safe, easy-to-find place in your home so you can grab one in a flash to take to an emergency department, then give copies to your pediatrician, your child's preferred hospital(s), your children's school, and all caregivers, relatives (including in-laws), babysitters, and friends whom your child spends time with when you're not around. It's a long list! Then make a list of this list so you remember who needs important updates.

Finally, put someone (probably *you*) in charge of updating the form periodically. After all, you can't choose when emergencies happen (though try your best to avoid Friday and Saturday nights!). But you can bet that you or your spouse won't be available at the precise moment your child becomes ill or is injured—and that even if you are, you won't be able to accurately recall some precious tidbit of medical info that could make all the difference when seconds count.

You can also find the form online—along with other helpful information about handling emergencies—at www.medical homeinfo.org/tools/emer_med.html (in both English and Spanish) and print it out. If possible, make copies on a machine that can enlarge originals so you don't need to write in microprint to squeeze everything in.

Working with the School

Some kids enjoy missing school—at least a day or two. Or three. But for children with chronic conditions, being out of school can become an unpleasant norm rather than an occasional treat. Missing classes, playtime, and school friends can further disrupt their life and make a tough time harder.

Make it a priority to work closely with your child's school. Meet with teachers, the principal, the counselor, the school nurse,

Emergency Information Form for Children With Special Needs

Last name:

American College of Emergency Physicians*	American Academy of Pediatrics	Date form completed	Revised	Initials
		By Whom	Revised	Initials

Name: | Birth date: | Nickname:

Home Address:	Home/Work Phone:
Parent/Guardian:	Emergency Contact Names & Relationship:
Signature/Consent*:	
Primary Language:	Phone Number(s):

Physicians:

Primary care physician:	Emergency Phone:
	Fax:
Current Specialty physician: Specialty:	Emergency Phone:
	Fax:
Current Specialty physician: Specialty:	Emergency Phone:
	Fax:
Anticipated Primary ED:	Pharmacy:
Anticipated Tertiary Care Center:	

Diagnoses/Past Procedures/Physical Exam:

1.	Baseline physical findings:
2.	
3.	Baseline vital signs:
4.	
Synopsis:	
	Baseline neurological status:

*Consent for release of this form to health care providers

(continued on next page)

Last name:

Diagnoses/Past Procedures/Physical Exam continued:

Medications: | Significant baseline ancillary findings (lab, x-ray, ECG):

1.

2.

3.

4. | Prostheses/Appliances/Advanced Technology Devices:

5.

6.

Management Data:

Allergies: Medications/Foods to be avoided and why:

1.

2.

3.

Procedures to be avoided and why:

1.

2.

3.

Immunizations

Dates						Dates					
DPT						Hep B					
OPV						Varicella					
MMR						TB status					
HIB						Other					

Antibiotic prophylaxis: Indication: Medication and dose:

Common Presenting Problems/Findings With Specific Suggested Managements

Problem | Suggested Diagnostic Studies | Treatment Considerations

Comments on child, family, or other specific medical issues:

Physician/Provider Signature: **Print Name:**

© American College of Emergency Physicians and American Academy of Pediatrics. Permission to reprint granted with acknowledgement.

Source: © American College of Emergency Physicans and American Academy of Pediatrics. Reprinted with permission. Available at http://www.medicalhomeinfo .org/tools/emer_med.html.

even the school secretary to explain your child's illness and how it might impact his schoolwork. See if your child's textbooks are available online.

As kids get older, many may not want the school to know about their medical condition. But tell your adolescent that the better informed the school staff is, the more they'll be to help him. As for his classmates, knowing what he's dealing with may reduce the chances that they'll tease, bully, or harass him—but that can be a *very* touchy subject, and your child needs to know that his confidence won't be betrayed if he doesn't want his classmates to know his private business. An older child needs to be given full control about what he's comfortable sharing with friends (or nonfriends), so talk it over but let him go from there. You can tell your child that his teachers and school staff will keep information confidential. His school should honor such requests.

It's really important that your child be involved with school activities as much as possible. Whenever there's an opportunity for a child with a chronic illness to act independently, support it to help their sense of self-esteem.

Although schools vary in the health assistance they offer, federal law requires public schools to provide chronically ill students with a "free and appropriate education in the least restrictive environment." Depending on your child's condition, those services include educational support, adaptive physical education, transportation, audiology, recreation, psychological services, physical and occupational therapy, speech and language therapy, assistive technology, and other help. If your child has special needs, the school should develop an Individualized Education Plan (IEP) for satisfying any medical requirements.

Coping Strategies

The hardest part of having a child with a serious illness or special needs may be **treating your child as normally as possible.**

Dealing with Bullies

If your child has a chronic condition, there's a chance that he'll be teased, mocked, or otherwise harassed by schoolyard peers (yes, children are still mean, despite all the "zero tolerance on teasing" programs that schools have launched in the last decade). He'll probably face aggressive behavior from bullies because he is "different"—unless "different" includes being a foot taller than his peers and a lot stronger. Remember that bullying can take many forms: name calling, ridiculing, being excluded from activities, and—thanks, technology—having cruel text messages or e-mails sent around about his condition. Of course, uncreative bullies still hit, kick, shove, and steal lunch money.

Obviously, children with conditions that affect their appearance (such as cerebral palsy, muscular dystrophy, or Down syndrome) are more likely to be victimized and called names. This can make these kids depressed, lonely, and anxious; ruin their self-confidence; trigger headaches, stomachaches, fatigue, and eating disorders; and make them *hate* school.

What can you do if your child is being bullied (by the way, it's called "disability harassment" in the eyes of the law)? Here's some advice from the U.S. Department of Health and Human Services' Stop Bullying Now campaign, which is targeted to children with special needs.

Be supportive, and encourage your child to describe who was involved and how and what happened. Don't encourage your child to fight back; that could make the problem worse. Usually, kids are able to tell you who bullied them, but some kids with disabilities don't realize that it may be a "friend" who's actually making fun of them. Know who your child's true friends are, and watch for bullies. Talk to your child's teacher, and if that doesn't fix the problem, see the principal and get your complaint down in writing. It may be helpful to also take the issue to the school district by scheduling a meeting with the Committee on Special Education (CSE) to talk about what the school is doing to stop the harassment and to spell out a plan in your child's Individualized Educational Plan (IEP).

It's a balancing act, for sure. While your child may require extra attention and care, you need to avoid going overboard. Emphasize your child's strengths—the things he can do well despite his condition. Some other family coping strategies:

- Keep the household routine as normal as possible.
- Remember that children do best when their daily routine is predictable and consistent, even though this won't always be possible given doctor's appointments, tests, flare-ups, or whatever else is on your plate.
- Prepare everyone in the family for any upcoming medical procedures your child may need by explaining what's being done, why, and how long it will take.
- Resist the temptation to coddle your child. It will be harder for him to participate in normal activities and may even create a relationship in which you both become needy and dependent on one another. Set limits and keep discipline consistent, which

will reassure him and provide all your children with structure and security.

- Encourage all family members to talk about their feelings. Remind each other that people everywhere are dealing with

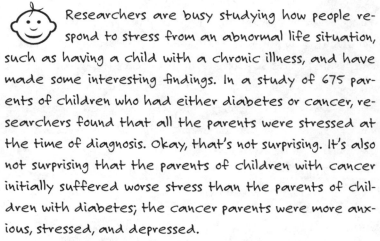

Stress Now vs. Stress Later

Researchers are busy studying how people respond to stress from an abnormal life situation, such as having a child with a chronic illness, and have made some interesting findings. In a study of 675 parents of children who had either diabetes or cancer, researchers found that all the parents were stressed at the time of diagnosis. Okay, that's not surprising. It's also not surprising that the parents of children with cancer initially suffered worse stress than the parents of children with diabetes; the cancer parents were more anxious, stressed, and depressed.

What is surprising, however, is what happened as time passed. The stress gradually diminished in the cancer parents but gradually *increased* in the diabetes group. Why? The researchers surmise that the children with cancer often were successfully treated, making the cancer less of a daily threat. But the children with diabetes—a lifelong, progressive illness—became more likely to develop problems.

The take-home? Make sure you practice stress-reducing strategies if your child has a long-term disability or chronic condition. I've included several effective suggestions in the sections below.

illnesses, disabilities, and challenges like the one your family is facing. Bring up some of the famous role models you've found (see page 126).

- Try to stay upbeat and positive. One psychologist who is an expert in dealing with chronically ill children tells families, "Eighty percent of what we worry about never happens." Keep that thought in the front of your brain.

Avoiding Relationship Problems

While many couples help each other get through their child's crisis, the frustration, guilt, exhaustion, and anger that hovers over parents during trying times can cause marriage troubles. The stress of caring for a chronically ill child can quickly bring any marital issues front and center.

One study found that parents of children with genetically based diseases, such as hemophilia, have a higher than 70 percent divorce rate. Having a sick child reminds a lot of parents of the first few months after childbirth, when exhaustion is the norm and there's virtually no time for sleep, recovery, or each other. The situation with a chronically ill child is the same thing but often with no end in sight. Normal outlets to recharge your batteries are hard to come by. You need to set up a support system and accept offers of help so that you and your spouse can find time for each other.

Depression: Worse in Moms?

It's not surprising that the parents of chronically ill children are often sad and upset about their child, but one study found that many moms display symptoms of severe depression and need some respite from their duties to decompress the pressure they feel as overloaded parents. The researchers examined 365 mothers whose children had a variety of conditions, such as asthma, sickle cell anemia, and heart disease. Symptoms of depression were high in the group as a whole, and 20 percent of the mothers felt that being a parent dominated their lives and restricted their freedom. More than half (59 percent) said their children were limited in their daily activities because of their illness. Researchers said that therapists and educators need to help mothers deal with feelings of anger and resentment. And as I've noted, support groups can be amazingly therapeutic, allowing strained-to-the-limit parents to verbalize what they're feeling about themselves and their child. Ask your doctor, school psychologist, or social worker if they know of any parent or family group that might be helpful to you. Also, contacting or visiting the websites of the organizations listed at the end of this chapter is another good place to start. If you don't want to join a support group, find one or two other parents who are facing similar challenges. Together, you can help each other through difficult times. Just knowing that someone else is experiencing similar successes and struggles can help relieve some of your stress.

Easing the Strain

When friends and family members offer to stay with your child or children so that you and your partner can enjoy a night out, find a way to say yes, even if you have to teach the person about medical equipment or drugs.

In New York, where I live, there's a directory of agencies, programs, and services such as day camps, child care, respite and after-school programs, health care, family support, parenting programs, counseling, and many other services. It's called "The Comprehensive Directory: Programs and Services for Children and Youth with Disabilities and Special Needs and Their Family in the Metro New York Area." The state also has the Office of Mental Retardation and Developmental Disabilities (OMRDD), which offers programs, services, and a resource directory. Your state probably has something similar. Just do an Internet search on "resources for children with special needs" along with the name of your state, and I bet several helpful options will surface. Other tips:

- Make sure you get enough rest.
- Pay attention to your spouse and talk about what you're both feeling.
- Don't plan ahead too much. Instead, break your child's treatment into small blocks of time so that you plan only for the next week or so.
- If you need help with the financial side of your child's illness, talk to your doctor or hospital staff about specific options for your child's condition.

Journaling or Blogging About Your Thoughts

You may not consider yourself a writer, but keeping a journal, diary, or blog allows you to put your thoughts and feelings into words and to discuss daily triumphs and trials. Your life has been drastically changed by your child's health. Some people do great venting in support groups, but others find it more therapeutic to write about their inner turmoil. You may start looking forward to having ten minutes every day or every week (or as often as you like) to just let it flow out of you. Find out more by going to www.specialchild.com and looking under "Family Issues." It's a useful website provided by the Resource Foundation for Children with Challenges, a not-for-profit organization.

Hello, Babysitter?

If you have a special-needs child, finding a good babysitter may seem totally impossible. But it's important to find time to re-connect with your partner or just go out with friends and see a movie or have dinner. So try this:

If possible, reach out to family first. They know your child (and vice versa) and are willing and able to deal with his special needs.

If that doesn't work, ask friends if they'll trade babysitting time with you so that there's no money involved and you can both pay back the favor.

Find out if there is a babysitting co-op in your neighborhood, especially through schools, day care, church, or early interven-tion classes.

Check with your child's school; there may be young teach-ers or aides who are looking to make a little extra money on the weekend. Or they may know of someone who is interested in babysitting and has experience dealing with chronically ill chil-dren.

Check the American Red Cross—it runs babysitting classes and may have a list of trained high school and college kids look-ing to earn extra money.

Traveling Tips

Fair or not (expect some sibling protests), family trips *have* to be planned around your special-needs child or odds are the trip will end in a health debacle, ruining it for everyone. Here are ways to ensure that the whole family has a blast.

- If your child has asthma, traveling to a warm and dry climate or a damp and cold one with salty air can help chronic breathing problems.

- If you're contemplating a long plane ride, be aware that pressurized cabins can create complications for children with respiratory, heart, or circulatory disorders. Make sure you check with your pediatrician or specialist beforehand.
- If you're traveling to a place like Disneyland, get a note from your doc explaining why your child can't stand in line for long periods of time to wait for an amusement park ride or exhibit. Often, special passes are available for children with special needs. (Check with guest services to find out.)
- If your child has diabetes and you're traveling across time zones, keep a written record of insulin or medication times to make sure your child's blood sugar remains constant. It's easy to get confused with time changes.
- On flights, take meds with you in a carry-on bag in case your luggage is lost or delayed.
- Since chronically ill children are more apt to need medical assistance on trips, check out which hospitals in your destination area are accredited by The Joint Commission. (If you're traveling domestically, go to www.jointcommission.org; for travel abroad, go to www.jointcommissioninternational.org.)

A CLOSER LOOK AT TWO INCREASINGLY COMMON CONDITIONS

Next, we'll take a closer look at autism and ADHD, two chronic conditions that commonly affect children.

The A-Word: Autism

Of all pediatric disorders, autism may be receiving the most attention today. Why? Because it's increasing rapidly among children for unknown reasons. I have a personal connection to this developmental disorder, as I've mentioned earlier. My oldest son, Noah, has autism. He's thirteen now, and the experiences I've had caring for him in the past decade have profoundly changed me as a parent, person, and pediatrician. I know the changes are for the better, and I think my patients know it, too. In some ways, my experiences with Noah have been even more influential to my practice than my medical school training and my practice prior to his diagnosis. Above all, his condition has instilled in me the ability to be more patient as a parent and more empathetic as a physician. I certainly better recognize and understand the added challenges a parent of a child with special needs faces on a daily basis. I also see things from a different perspective than other pediatricians—I see things from the perspective of a parent of a child with special needs.

What Is Autism Spectrum Disorder (ASD)?

For starters, it's not one disorder. It's several. Simply broken down, ASD includes a range of neurological and developmental impairments that affect how individuals interact socially, communicate verbally and nonverbally, think, learn, move, and play. An estimated 1 in 150 children falls somewhere within the autism spectrum. (See appendix B for more information about the individual disorders that make up the autism spectrum.) In most cases, the cause is unknown—however, there is a strong genetic component. Continued biological and environmental research is needed to understand what triggers most autism.

Traditional and Alternative Treatments for Autism

My first recommendation with any childhood health issue is always to work closely with your pediatrician. (Shocking advice from me, right?) Many of us have specific training and practical experience caring for autistic and other special-needs children. We will recommend the best treatments for your child and help you evaluate the scientific merits of all therapies. By the way,

FACT: Most often, children with an autistic spectrum disorder (ASD) are diagnosed by the time they're three.

FACT: Although autism disorders don't occur in any one race or culture more than another, they do have a gender bias: Autism affects four times as many boys as girls.

early intervention is very important. If your pediatrician doesn't seem to have a sense of urgency about helping your child, look for a pediatrician who specializes in ASD.

My second recommendation is **don't get lured in by treatments that claim to cure autism.** There is no known cure.

So what can help? Educational approaches, such as applied behavioral analysis (or ABA), which has become widely accepted as an effective treatment and is backed up by scientific evidence. Educational approaches are the cornerstone for treating any form of autism, and they include teaching autistic kids, many hours per week, the social, academic, and daily living skills that most children acquire naturally; providing speech, language, and occupational therapy; and generally minimizing the kinds of behaviors that make autistic kids stand out and instilling patterns that help them fit in and function independently.

Sometimes medications help, too, by easing difficult symptoms, especially aggressive or obsessive behavior, or helping to relieve anxiety.

What about special diets? I'd be very careful with anything that involves what your child eats. For example, the gluten-free/casein-free diet, often touted as an alternative treatment for autism, increases the risk of rickets, a bone disease caused by a vitamin D/calcium deficiency. The diet eliminates dairy foods—a key source of calcium and D—and parents do not always give their children enough supplements to make up for missing these nutrients in meals. Rickets softens bones and may lead to deformities and fractures.

It is vital to *work closely with your doctor.* If you have questions or are curious about a new therapy, ask about it. Together, you can start with traditional therapies and, if you and your doctor choose to, carefully add complementary alternative treatments to see if any of them help—keeping in mind that each child is different and not everything will be effective on all children. Here's a smart way to approach whether a specific treatment might be worth trying on your child.

1. **How good is the evidence for it?** Your doctor can help you weigh this. One aspect to consider: Is the evidence based on scientific research or is it anecdotal?
2. **How safe is it?** With music therapy, there's unlikely to be any risk. With major diet changes or drugs, the risk is much higher.
3. **How expensive is it?** Is a music therapist or acupuncturist even available in your area? Will regular treatments require significant time/money sacrifices from other members of the family? Are they game for this?
4. **What do you think the benefits will be?** Are there specific symptoms you hope to see improved, or are the reputed benefits pretty vague?

Finally, try one treatment at a time to evaluate its effectiveness, and be aware of what your child's abilities are when you start. And remember, autism tends to have ups and downs, with bursts of improvement mixed with times of slower learning or even periods of regression. Because of this variability, it may be difficult to establish a cause and effect for a given treatment.

For information on where to go for help and support, you'll find a list of resources at the end of this chapter.

Attention Deficit/Hyperactivity Disorder (ADHD)

Attention deficit/hyperactivity disorder (ADHD) is running a close second behind autism for media coverage and parental worry today. It's so commonly diagnosed that somewhere between 5 and 10 percent of children have it, depending on which statistics you believe. That could mean up to four million children in the United States—predominantly boys, who are three times more susceptible to it than girls—have ADHD. What's most important about ADHD is that it directly impacts your child's ability to function at home and at school, because it is characterized by inattentiveness, overactivity, impulsivity, or a combination of these.

Sure, at times *all* kids have trouble focusing, act without thinking, and can be hyperactive. The difference with ADHD is that symptoms last for at least six months, are more severe than in other kids the same age, and occur in two areas of the child's life, usually at home and in school. A child with ADHD may understand what's expected of him, but he has trouble following through because he can't pay attention, sit still, or listen to details. To be officially diagnosed, the disruptive behaviors cannot be linked to upsetting events such as a divorce, a move, a severe illness, or a change in schools, because those stressors may cause your child to act out for an extended period of time.

There are actually three types of ADHD: inattentive, hyperactive-impulsive, and combined, which is the most common. Most cases are diagnosed by a pediatrician, but there's no single test for the disorder. The diagnosis is made after a complete physical exam, an extensive medical history, and a long talk with your doctor about what you've been noticing at home. And that's not all. Next, your doctor will talk to your child's teachers (and a school psychologist, if there is one) and ask them to make observations and fill out questionnaires and rating scales. (Many teachers are achingly familiar with this drill.) That information gathering will also help evaluate possible coexisting concerns, such as a learning disability, depression, or an anxiety disorder.

What Causes ADHD?

One of the first questions a parent will ask me is "What did I do wrong? Did I cause this?" There is no evidence that ADHD is caused by lapses in child rearing, reactions to vaccines, or giving in to countless requests for sugar-loaded cookies. I tell parents to forget their inner blame game and focus on finding the best possible way to help their child. Let researchers try to discover the cause for ADHD.

And they're trying hard. Scientists believe genetic and environmental factors may play a role, and studies show that many children with ADHD have a close relative who also has the disorder. Experts also know that kids with ADHD have chemical changes in their brain and that certain areas of the brain are about 5 to 10 percent smaller in size and activity than normal.

Other studies about the cause of ADHD point to links with smoking during pregnancy, premature delivery, very low birth weight, and injuries to the brain at birth. Some research suggests a link between excessive early TV watching and attention issues. (That's one of the reasons the AAP says that children under two should not have any screen time—that means no computers, TV, DVDs, or video games—and that kids two and older should watch no more than one to two hours a day of nonviolent, quality TV.)

About two-thirds of children with ADHD also have other problems, such as depression, anxiety, dyslexia, or trouble writing. About 35 percent of all children with ADHD have oppositional defiant disorder, which makes them extremely stubborn, defiant, and aggressive and causes them to throw tantrums. It's thought that about 25 percent of children with ADHD have anxiety disorders in which they have excessive worry, fear, or panic.

Treating ADHD

While ADHD can't be cured, it can be managed with a combination of drugs and behavioral therapy. It sounds odd, but a class of medications known as stimulants has been used for more than fifty years to help ADHD. Nonstimulants and antidepressants are also options. But it's impossible to predict which will help or whether your child will react badly to some of them. Not all children respond to the first medicine prescribed to them—and many come with side effects—so don't be discouraged if you need to try several different meds to find one that works for your kid. The goal is to decrease the ADHD symptoms without causing unwanted side effects.

Make sure your doctor specializes in ADHD and has a lot of experience. Medications should always be taken in the lowest dose possible that produces the desired results—this will minimize side effects. The dose should start low and, if necessary, be increased slowly under the watchful eye of your doctor. Medicine for ADHD only controls the symptoms and only on the day it is taken, but it will help your child pay better attention and complete schoolwork. About 80 percent of children who need medication for ADHD still need it as teenagers, and about 50 percent need it as adults.

Behavioral therapy includes setting up a system of rewards for positive behavior to help children build self-esteem. To me, behavior management therapy is almost always beneficial because your child will learn how to be better organized and how to break down large tasks into smaller, manageable pieces with the help of timetables and schedules. Many schools have developed special programs to help kids with ADHD. While there is no specific cure for ADHD, a long-term management plan will help bring encouraging results.

Depending on the severity, your doctor may recommend behavioral therapy, medication, or a combination of the two. To help you and your child cope, you can also try parent training, which teaches you how to help your child with ADHD (and helps you cope with it too). The National Institutes of Health has a good website where you can find more help: health.nih.gov/ topic/AttentionDeficitHyperactivityDisorder. There's also a list of organizations that may be of help at www.nih.gov.disorders/

adhd.htm. You'll find a more complete list of resources at the end of this chapter.

WAYS TO COPE

* Keep to the same routine every day, from early morning until bedtime. Include set times for play and homework, and post the schedule in a prominent place so your child can see it.
* Help your child organize everyday items, such as clothing, backpacks, and school supplies. Keep everything in the same place.
* Use notebooks and organizers to make sure your child writes down homework assignments and brings home needed books and supplies.
* Remember to praise your child. Children with ADHD receive a lot of criticism, so look for good behavior and hand out gold stars whenever it happens (yes, gold stars still work).
* Ask your child's teacher to provide feedback to your child in private and to avoid asking your child to do a task in front of others that might be too difficult for him.

Some parents try alternative therapies, such as large doses of vitamins, Chinese herbals, or iron supplements, and report improvements in their children. You should know that cutting out all white sugar from your child's diet has not been shown to do a bit of good (except for their teeth). However, a small study recently suggested that eliminating food preservatives may help, but no large-scale study has proven that. Still, if you want to try this, I would recommend eliminating just one additive at a time to see if you notice any difference.

Additional Resources

In addition to your doctors, help, support, and information about special needs and chronic illnesses are plentiful. Resources range from websites to chat rooms filled with parents like you and me, sharing daily successes and struggles. Check out these resources for more information on common conditions and chronic illnesses.

ADHD
AD/HD Global Network
www.global-adhd.org/
Attention Deficit Disorder Association
www.add.org

Centers for Disease Control and Prevention home page for ADHD
www.cdc.gov/ncbddd/adhd/index.html

Children and Adults with Attention Deficit/Hyperactivity Disorder
www.chadd.org

National Institute of Mental Health
www.nimh.nih.gov/

National Resource Center on AD/HD
www.help4adhd.org

Asthma
American Academy of Allergy Asthma and Immunology
(414) 272-6071
www.aaaai.org

American Lung Association
(800) LUNG-USA
www.lungusa.org

Asthma and Allergy Foundation of America
(800) 7-ASTHMA
www.aafa.org

Autism
American Academy of Pediatrics autism page
www.aap.org/healthtopics/autism.cfm

Asperger Syndrome Education Network
www.aspennj.org

Association for Science in Autism Treatment
www.asatonline.org

AutismAsperger.net

Autism Online
www.autismonline.com

Autism Science Foundation
www.autismsciencefoundation.org

Autism Society
www.autism-society.org

Autism Speaks
www.autismspeaks.org

Closing the Gap (assistive technology resources for children and adults with special needs)
www.closingthegap.com

First Signs
www.firstsigns.org

Future Horizons
www.fhautism.com

Interactive Autism Network
www.iancommunity.org

National Dissemination Center for Children with Disabilities
www.nichcy.org

Cancer
American Cancer Society
(800) ACS-2345
www.cancer.org

National Cancer Institute
(800) 4-CANCER
www.cancer.gov

National Comprehensive Cancer Network
(215) 690-0300
www.nccn.com

Cerebral Palsy
National Institute of Neurological Disorders and Stroke at the
National Institutes of Health
(800) 352-9424
www.ninds.nih.gov/disorders/cerebral_palsy

Pathways Awareness (for children with movement difficulties)
www.pathwaysawareness.org
(800) 955-2445

Pedal-with-Pete (research on cerebral palsy)
(800) 304-7383
www.pedalwithpete.com

United Cerebral Palsy (UCP)
(800) 872-5827
www.ucp.org

Congenital Heart Problems
American Heart Association
(800) AHA-USA1
www.americanheart.org

Congenital Heart Information Network
(215) 627-4034
tchin.org

Mended Little Hearts
(888) HEART99
mendedhearts.org/mlh/frame-mlh.htm

Cystic Fibrosis
Cystic Fibrosis Foundation
(800) FIGHT-CF
www.cff.org

March of Dimes
(914) 997-4488
www.marchofdimes.com

Diabetes
American Diabetes Association
(800) DIABETES
www.diabetes.org/for-parents-and-kids.jsp

Juvenile Diabetes Research Foundation International
(800) 533-CURE
www.jdrf.org/index.cfm

National Diabetes Education Program at the National Institutes
for Health
(301) 496-3583
www.ndep.nih.gov/index.aspx

Down Syndrome
National Association for Down Syndrome
(630) 325-9112
www.nads.org

National Down Syndrome Society
(800) 221-4602
www.ndss.org

National Institute on Developmental Delays
(405) 878-5289
www.nidd.org

Dyslexia and Learning Disabilities
International Dyslexia Association
(410) 296-0232
www.interdys.org

Learning Disabilities Association of America
(412) 341-1515
www.ldaamerica.org

National Center for Learning Disabilities
(888) 575-7373
www.ld.org

Epilepsy
Epilepsy.com
(540) 687-8077
www.epilepsy.com/kids/kids

Epilepsy Foundation
(800) 332-1000
www.epilepsyfoundation.org

Kidney Disease
National Kidney and Urologic Diseases Information
Clearinghouse
(800) 891-5390
kidney.niddk.nih.gov/index.htm

National Kidney Foundation
(800) 622-9010
www.kidney.org/kidneydisease/parents.cfm

Liver Disease
American Association for the Study of Liver Diseases
(703) 299-9766
publish.aasld.org/Pages/Default.aspx

American Liver Foundation
(212) 668-1000
www.liverfoundation.org

Mental Retardation
American Academy of Child and Adolescent Psychiatry
(202) 966-7300
www.aacap.org/cs/root/facts_for_families/children_who_are
_mentally_retarded

American Association on Intellectual and Developmental
Disabilities
(800) 424-3688
www.aamr.org

Sickle Cell Anemia
Save Babies Through Screening Foundation
(888) 454-3383
www.savebabies.org

Sickle Cell Disease Association of America
(800) 421-8453
www.sicklecelldisease.org

Spina Bifida
National Dissemination Center for Children with Disabilities
(800) 695-0285
www.nichcy.org

Spina Bifida Association
(800) 621-3141
www.sbaa.org

CHAPTER 4 POP QUIZ ANSWERS

1. How many U.S. children between the ages of two and eighteen are estimated to have a chronic health problem? The answer is C, about 30 percent. (Page 114.)

2. What does "CSHCN" stand for? The answer is B, "children with special health care needs." (Page 115.)

3. Which of these statements about asthma is true? The answer is B—asthma becomes inactive in about half of kids when they hit their teens. (Page 120.)

4. Which of these statements about attention deficit/hyperactivity disorder (ADHD) is true? The answer is C—about 50 percent will still need medication when they're adults. (Page 149.)

5. Which of these historical figures is thought to have had ADHD? The answer is B, Galileo, although Howdy Doody did seem to lose focus pretty often. (Page 126.)

Chapter 5

When Should You Absolutely, Positively Rush to the ER?

How to Get Seen Fast

POP QUIZ

Do you know what to do in an emergency? Do you know what's *really* an emergency versus what could be handled in a doctor's office? If you can answer all of the following questions correctly (there may be more than one correct choice)—and you're gutsy—then you can skip this chapter. Check your answers at the end of the chapter and see how well you did. Good luck!

1. How do you find the best ED or urgent care facility for your child?
   A. Drive fast in what you think is the right direction, with your screaming child next to you, and pray you spot a blue "hospital" sign.
   B. Dial 911 and let the paramedics select one for you.
   C. Before an emergency strikes, find an ED that is in a Joint Commission–accredited hospital, or a facility that is Joint Commission accredited, and equipped to treat children.
   D. If they're on the evening news a lot, they must be good!

2. How do you know if it's really an emergency?
   A. Your aunt Agnes says so (she goes to the ED for sore throats).
   B. Your heartbeat is racing, and you feel faint. Your child's not doing so well either.

C. Your gut tells you this is the real deal and you need to get help fast.

D. Your craving for chocolate won't subside.

3. When is it okay to drive to the ED?

    A. When you are not hyperventilating over the sight of your child's blood

    B. When your car has plenty of gas and two adults in it

    C. When your mother-in-law says you shouldn't

    D. When your child does not have a head, neck, or back injury, is awake and responding, and is breathing without problems

4. What's the secret for getting fast service in the ED?

    A. Having a bad flu and throwing up in a crowded waiting room

    B. Telling the triage nurse she reminds you of Miss USA

    C. Bringing a box of fresh, chewy brownies with you

    D. Being super nice to the staff and asking your pediatrician to call ahead

5. How do you find out if your local hospital's ED is kid friendly?

    A. Ask the neighborhood bully, who's been there several times.

    B. Talk to your doctor and do some research.

    C. Ask your ninety-five-year-old grandmother what she thinks.

    D. Go to the ED and poll everyone in the waiting room.

6. What should you do if your toddler swallows a pink Barbie shoe?

    A. Call the doctor, and if you're told to come in or go to the ED, bring the shoe's mate with you.

    B. Cry and call your best friend for advice.

    C. Tell Barbie's owner (your older daughter) not to leave her toys lying around on the floor.

    D. If your child is not choking, things will likely be just fine.

7. Should you stay with your child in the ED, even when he goes for tests?

    A. Yes, always

    B. A smile, a warm cuddle, and holding hands can't hurt

    C. Yes, unless you're squeamish or get ill at the thought of certain procedures, like blood draws.

    D. All of the above

8. Will your kids ever grow up and stop having accidents and getting sick in the middle of the night?

    A. No, not until they are thirty-five or so. Perhaps even later.

    B. Yes, when you least expect it

    C. Uh-huh, when you're in the retirement home or Sun City

    D. It's called being a parent. Get used to it.

So, the kids are doing fine?

    Couldn't be better?

    Fantastic. Now's the time to think about the day when they won't be. Do you have a plan for when your six-year-old, rushing down a flight of stairs, falls and hits her head? She's screaming, your heart is racing, her forehead is sprouting an enormous goose egg, and . . . well, can it get any better than this? Do you call the pediatrician? Dial 911? Or scoop up your child, grab an ice bag, and drive like a crazy person to the nearest emergency room?

    If you don't have a clue, I empathize. Through the years, many people have heard conflicting advice about using emergency rooms. And when it seems like everything is falling to pieces, and your child is screaming, writhing, and possibly getting blood all over the hallway carpet, your brain isn't exactly functioning at its best. You need to make decisions fast—and hope that they're the right ones.

    That's why you need to make those decisions now, *before* an emergency strikes. Then you'll know they'll be right, and you won't have to rely on hasty guesswork in a situation when every second might count. Or a situation in which a seemingly small decision—such as heading left to the county general hospital rather than right to that big medical center a bit farther away (or vice versa)—could mean years of regret.

What Are the Odds?

One out of every 2.4 children will be seen in an emergency department this year. That means your chances of making that trip are high, even if you're the most super-careful parent. Kids are patients in about one-quarter of all emergency department visits. Think of it as a parenting rite of passage that includes a $200 copay.

That trip could come at any moment, triggered by a kid's ear-splitting headache, a bad cut, a broken bone, a breathing problem, or a seizure. Or—brace yourself—a lacerated tongue. That last one was added to my own personal list a few years ago when my then-eight-year-old son took a bad fall and in the process nearly cut his tongue off. He was in excruciating pain.

Now, I knew which emergency department was best equipped to handle most childhood injuries. But this wasn't most childhood injuries; it was a serious tongue laceration. And I also knew that this particular ED didn't have a pediatric anesthesiologist on-site. So instead of taking him there, I quickly called a nearby pediatric oral surgeon's office in the desperate hope that he was free to handle an immediate emergency—and, fortunately, he was. My son needed twenty deep stitches under general anesthesia (IV sedation plus a breathing tube). The next dozen hours weren't nearly as bad as they could have been for my son . . . and me.

From my personal example, you can see that sometimes the best emergency care isn't at the emergency room.

Of course, I was fortunate. As a pediatrician, I knew that general anesthesia would be critical for my son's treatment. But as a smart parent I had already made it my business to know how well the local emergency departments were equipped to treat pediatric pain. In those moments when I had to dial one number or another, that knowledge was invaluable. And it's available to every parent who seeks it.

Ten Ways to Keep Your Child Out of the Emergency Department

1. Talk to your pediatrician before giving any over-the-counter meds to children ages two and younger. Call your doctor, too, before you give cold or cough meds to children under five, and remember to keep the meds out of their reach. More than seven thousand children are rushed to the ED every year for bad reactions to cough and cold medicines, according to the Centers for Disease Control and Prevention. (That includes a lot of kids who guzzled the stuff without their parents' knowledge, so keep it locked up.)

2. Make sure your kids wear helmets and other protective gear for biking, in-line skating, skateboarding, and other sports. Roller shoes alone contributed to 1,600 emergency department visits in just one year, the Consumer Product Safety Commission reports.

3. Since a small child can drown in only a few inches of water, install locks on your toilet bowl lids, and never leave a bucket or container with water in it unattended, much less a bathtub or swimming pool. An adult must always be present around water. Period.

4. Burns from scalding water are a very common ED injury, so make sure your water heater's thermostat is set below 120 degrees. And keep curling irons, clothing irons, and steaming cups of coffee out of reach of little ones.

5. Watch those electrical outlets. Keep cords hidden from view so that toddlers are not tempted to chew on them. Put furniture in front of outlets with plugs in them.

6. Falls are another common reason for trips to the ED. If you have a second floor, keep those windows closed and locked or protect them with safety bars. If furniture can be climbed on, don't put it near a window. In homes with young kids, safety gates should be at the top and bottom of every flight of stairs. Never, ever leave a baby on a bed or changing table, even if you have pillows around the infant. Babies are *excellent* rollers. You wouldn't believe how many babies are hurt in preventable accidents because well-meaning parents didn't think their babies could roll so far.

7. Keep all dangerous cleaners, paint thinners, antifreeze, pesticides, and medicines locked up or on high shelves. Ditto for mouthwash, perfumes, vitamins, laundry detergent, and batteries—all can be deadly poisons to small kids, so make sure they are not accessible.

8. Recheck your home for choking hazards. Tip: If an object can fit in a cardboard toilet-paper tube, it's a choking hazard. Do a clean sweep and make sure all small objects are out of both sight and reach of young ones. Tie up cords from blinds and drapery, and keep ropes, ribbons, string, and plastic grocery bags away from small children.

9. Stow first-aid kits in your home and in every car in the family. Make sure your children and caretakers know where they are, and once your children are old enough, teach them about first aid.

10. Take a course in pediatric first aid that includes cardiopulmonary resuscitation (CPR) and the Heimlich maneuver. Find out more at www.redcross.org.

Make an Emergency Plan

Step one in being prepared for an emergency involves—guess who?—your pediatrician. If you haven't already done so, ask how your doctor prefers to deal with emergencies so you're prepared when the spaghetti hits the fan. The American College of Emergency Physicians says only one out of five families with kids discusses emergencies with their doctor—which is probably a big reason why only one-third of parents say they feel prepared to handle a real emergency.

Here are the six core questions to ask your child's doc, along with some follow-ups for each. We'll look more closely at these in the pages ahead.

1. **Should I call you before or during any trip to the emergency department?** The answer should be an unequivocal yes—or you need a new pediatrician (see page 69). Maybe you'll find out the trip isn't necessary. Maybe your doctor will want to meet you there. Maybe your doctor will remind you about what to tell the ED doc. Also, some insurance plans require a doctor's preauthorization before an ED visit for conditions that are usually not true emergencies.

2. **What's the best, quickest way to reach you or your backup team after office hours?** Again, if these answers aren't up to par, you need to find a new pediatrician before an emergency strikes.

3. **Will you call ahead to expedite my child's care once I arrive?** In almost every case, your pediatrician will be able to grease the wheels once you get to the ED. Even when I've been traveling several states away, I've often gotten my patients to the front of the ED line (when there's been good reason) because they called me and I called the ED. Also, I often talk to parents on the phone while their child is in the ED about what tests will likely be performed, what the

diagnosis may be, and what treatment options to expect. The ED docs don't have time to talk this through with parents while they're working on their child, so many parents find it comforting to be clued in on what's going on (or what's likely going on, anyway) and what amusements are coming next.

4. **What hospital do you prefer for pediatric emergencies?** Does your doc have full privileges there? Can the hospital doctors get access to your child's complete medical record and health history? Also find out if the ED staff includes pediatric emergency medicine physicians, which means they've received extra training in handling childhood traumas.

5. **If the emergency is not life threatening, is there an urgent care center that you recommend?**

6. **What else do I need to know? Is there anything I should bring with me if I go to the ED? Is there anything I should be especially concerned about if my child is having a medical emergency?**

Find the Right Emergency Department

That mammoth city hospital about sixteen miles from your home may be "world renowned," offer the absolute best emergency care in a hundred-mile radius, and even have the spiffiest cafeteria known to medical science.

So why could it be a bad choice for your child?

Because kids—especially when they're younger than ten—need to be treated in emergency departments that are specially designed and equipped to treat little bodies. Yes, sometimes speed is crucial, and then any medical care is always (well, almost always) better than none. But in the vast majority of cases, taking your child to a well-equipped pediatric emergency department is much safer and wiser than opting for a closer ED that doesn't cater to children. And there's more to that than having wallpaper with duckies.

Shockingly, even though children make up 27 percent of all ED visits, 94 percent of hospitals in the United States do not have all the necessary supplies for pediatric emergencies, according to a study by the Institute of Medicine. One hospital reported it didn't have child-sized neck braces, so the ED staff used rolled-up towels to stabilize children's spines. Did that make you wince? It made *me* wince.

What's more, some 85 percent of the beds and equipment in most hospitals are designed for adults. That's also not good, as small kids can roll under adult-bed handrails and hit the floor. Other reports found that some hospitals had only adult-sized oxygen masks, which are too big for a child's face and wouldn't effectively deliver oxygen to a kid having a severe asthma attack.

Shortcomings like these persist among many hospitals despite standards and regulations meant to prevent them. The American Academy of Pediatrics has minimum requirements for equipment, supplies, and medicine that should be available in any ED that treats children. The list is long, and it includes pediatric-sized blood pressure devices, stethoscopes, oxygen masks, chest tubes, butterfly needles, infant scales, splints, and more. Seeing the words "Pediatric Emergency Department" on the hospital's double doors is no guarantee that the ED is up to standard.

So how can you find the best pediatric emergency department in your area? Ask your pediatrician, of course, but do some detective work, too. Start by calling or stopping by an ED to speak with the hospital's director of emergency services and asking these questions:

1. Do you have a pediatric emergency care specialist on staff— or at least pediatricians available 24/7? About 40 percent of EDs in the U.S. don't even have round-the-clock access to pediatricians, according to the Centers for Disease Control and Prevention. You want to be sure that *your* child's ED is staffed with pediatricians, pediatric nurses, and ideally, pediatric emergency medicine specialists (not just general emergency physicians). If it is, in my experience it's the strongest indication that they'll have the right equipment that you need in a pediatric ED.

2. Do you have medications in doses appropriate for children? Are they available in liquid forms or chewables? This is important. Many hospitals don't have pediatric medications, and it can cause life-threatening complications. Here's a common example: Recently, one of my patients—a toddler with asthma—had a sudden onset of respiratory distress. Unfortunately, his mother didn't call me and went straight to a hospital that didn't have a pediatric ED. He needed to take an oral steroid to control his symptoms, so the doctors crushed adult tabs for him. Not surprisingly, he kept spitting them out. Given how horribly bitter they must have tasted, I can't blame him. In the end, the toddler didn't get the dosage he needed, which probably hindered his recovery. His mother did bring him to see me in the morning, though, and I was able to give him the appropriate medicine then.

3. Does your ED have child-sized resuscitation equipment? Are there beds, IVs, and oxygen masks made for children? They need to be well stocked in extra-smalls.

4. Do you have a separate area just for pediatric patients? A good pediatric ED will have a kid-friendly section that will look more like a Chuck E. Cheese restaurant than an acute medical care facility. You should find a TV, cartoon DVDs, a few toys, and coloring books (though try to remember to bring comforting favorites from home, too). While the distractions are helpful, here's the real benefit: Your child will be shielded from the drama in the average ED and won't have to watch people arriving with heart attacks, gushing blood, or knife wounds. As a bonus, neither will you. Germ-wise, stress-wise, and sanity-wise, this is better for everybody.

Unfortunately, many hospitals don't have a special emergency area for children, which means your four-year-old could be sitting next to an inebriated guy who just shot a .22 bullet into his foot and is not happy about it.

5. How many children under age five do you treat every week? More than fifty is a good answer; three is not. You want an ED staff that's adept in dealing with screaming babies, frantic toddlers, and—not that you'll personally need this angle of their expertise, of course—hysterical parents.

6. Do you have a separate urgent-care satellite center? If a nearby hospital doesn't have a dedicated pediatric ED, at least

Green Acres, but No General Hospital?

If you live in a rural area where the best hospital to treat your child is eighty miles away, you may have few choices nearby. But now some local hospitals are using telemedicine to consult with pediatric specialists at large city hospitals via phone and video connections. Physicians call a toll-free number and are connected with a specialist in pediatric emergency care within minutes. And many children's hospitals are opening off-site pediatric emergency rooms in community hospitals, because parents are asking for those specialized services closer to home. Contact the emergency or pediatric department at your local hospital to see if they provide any of these services.

you're likely to get treated faster in the satellite center than the general ED. Similarly, the ED will be less crowded with non-life-threatening cases due to the satellite center.

7. Is the hospital accredited by The Joint Commission? If so, it means the hospital has voluntarily met national health and safety standards. You don't need to interrogate an ED staffer to find this out; you can learn if the hospital is accredited (as well as how it's performing in several key areas) at www.qualitycheck .org.

8. Are there Spanish and/or other translators on-site? You may speak English, but—and this is a big point that many people dangerously overlook—does your child's nanny, babysitter, or grandparent-who-watches-her-every-day speak English? Believe me, this can be critical. When your mother-in-law is on a cell phone with a bad connection and I have to rely on what I remem-

---

Know Before You Go

Kids have a penchant for having accidents on trips, thanks to unfamiliar surroundings and the opportunity to play on the slippery rocks after you've told them not to eleven times. So when taking a child on vacation, the most important bit of trip research you do could be scouting out the nearest and best ED at your destination area beforehand. And it's easy. Just go to www.qualitycheck.org to find hospitals that have been accredited by The Joint Commission in any U.S. location, or check out www.jointcommissioninternational.org to find accredited international organizations.

ber from French 101 to decipher what she's telling me about your son's bike accident and medication allergies, no one is happy.

Once you've identified your best emergency option, map out how to get there and do a couple of dry runs *before* you actually have a crying little one gushing blood in your backseat. In a real emergency, you might not be driving—you might not even be in your own vehicle—but at least you'll know how to get there. Someday, that might also help you decide whether to drive yourself and your child to the ED or to call 911.

But don't throw away your list of other choices. If an emergency strikes when your daughter is at a sleepover four towns away or your son is playing Little League in a neighboring community, it may come in handy. Unfortunately, by their very nature, emergencies are unplanned. Be prepared. Have backups.

Is It *Really* an Emergency?

A pediatric emergency is any unforeseen, sudden situation *during which you truly believe* that your child needs immediate medical care to prevent an illness or injury from potentially causing permanent harm or even death.

In other words, it's what your gut tells you during a crisis and the judgment you make about a situation *while it's happening*. Who are *you*? You're a reasonable, sane, normal average person—or what the American College of Emergency Physicians and the American health care system call a "prudent layperson."

Why is the emphasis on what you think while the situation is happening important here? Because a bout of mysterious, severe stomach pain is a "medical emergency" for your eleven-year-old (and for your health insurer) even if you spend thirteen hours in an ER and run up a $17,000 bill for tests, only to find out later that he was just a little gassy. You're not expected to know the difference between potentially fatal appendicitis and a bad tummy-ache; that's a doctor's job.

Always Call 911 If Your Child Has Any of These Signs

If your child has any of these signs, you're facing a life-threatening medical emergency. Call 911 and use an ambulance. You should also call your pediatrician while you're en route to the hospital, or have someone else call.

* A laceration (wound or cut) that is deep or large or involves the chest, head, or abdomen
* A large burn that involves the hands, face, or groin
* Evidence that your child has swallowed a poisonous substance or medication
* Confusion, headache, vomiting, or loss of consciousness after a head injury
* Uncontrollable seizures
* Severe respiratory distress and/or skin or lips that look blue, purple, or gray (bright red skin and lips usually aren't a serious problem)
* Loss of consciousness or syncope—the medical term for fainting.

Call Your Pediatrician If Your Infant (Under One Year) Has Any of These Signs

These are danger signs that need attention fast. If you can't reach your child's doctor quickly, get your child to the ED or an urgent care center right away. Ditto if your pediatrician doesn't think it's an emergency but you still have strong doubts. **When in doubt, always head to the emergency department or urgent care center.**

* Inconsolable crying or lethargy
* Vomiting and/or diarrhea for twenty-four hours or more
* Dry diapers for twelve hours or more
* Difficulty breathing
* Refusing fluids for twenty-four hours or more
* A fever above 100.4 degrees (taken rectally) in infants less than two months old
* Fever with a red or purple rash
* Seizure-like jerking movements
* General listlessness, dry mouth, crying with no tears, not urinating or urinating very dark urine (all signs of dehydration; see page 181 for more info).

Signs of Serious Illness in Children Ages One or Older (and Adults of *All* Ages)

These warning signs of severe illness should set off your "red alert" button and prompt a call to your pediatrician or doctor. They are often (but not always) medical emergencies that must be treated right away.

* Abdominal pain
* Difficulty breathing
* Severe headache or neck pain
* Increasing trouble breathing or chest pain
* General listlessness, dry mouth, crying with no tears, not urinating, or urinating very dark urine (all signs of dehydration; see page 181 for more info)
* Loss of consciousness or syncope—the medical term for fainting.

This means that rule number one in deciding whether your child is having a true emergency—and needs to go to the ED *now*, not to your pediatrician's office in a few hours or tomorrow—is the little voice in your head that says, "This is bad, and I can see it getting worse real quick."

What to Bring with You

The paramedics are on their way, or you are heading to the car to drive to the emergency department with your slightly hysterical daughter, who just took a nasty spill on her bike.

Rewind! Before you leave, grab your daughter's family medical history form, which you have handy just for such occasions. Are you thinking, "I don't have one of those, Dr. Jen?" No problem. Because you are reading this book and *not* on your way to the ED at this very moment, you have time to get this together. Please do so as soon as possible so you're prepared for an emergency. When you get to the ED, the nurses and doctors will need to know your child's medical history before they give her anything for her condition. Some medications don't mix well or there may be allergic reactions they need to know about, so having them listed on a sheet of paper that the docs can peruse quickly will help expedite the care. You'll be surprised how your mind can go blank in an emergency.

This medical form should include your child's current height and weight (preferably in kilograms), food or drug allergies, immunizations, past illnesses, injuries, surgeries, and any chronic conditions. If your child takes any medications, the medical record should list these drugs and dosages. For example, if your child has diabetes or asthma, you'll need to tell the paramedics and the emergency docs exactly when your child last had her meds and the dosages because both can have a big impact on the tests and treatment given at the hospital. You may think this will all come to you in a moment of heart-stomping panic, but it may not. And having all this information written down in front of them may help the doctors do a better, quicker job of diagnosing your child during an emergency. Their trained eyes may spot something about your child's current condition and relate it to her past, which may bring an *a-ha!* moment in their diagnosis.

Having a written medical record at home is also handy for

Poison

If your child **swallows poison:** If you find your child with an open or empty container of anything that isn't food, he may have eaten something poisonous. Stay calm and act quickly.

* First, get the item away from your child. If there is still some in his mouth, make him spit it out or remove it with your fingers. Keep this material along with any other clues about what your child ate.
* Save the container to help doctors determine exactly what and how much was swallowed.
* If your child is unconscious, not breathing, having convulsions, or having seizures, call 911 right away.
* If your child does not have these symptoms, call the poison center at 1-800-222-1222 (see the "Poison Hotline" box below). If the poison is very dangerous or your child is very young, you may be told to go straight to the nearest hospital. If not, you will be asked for the following information and told what to do at home.
  * Your name and phone number
  * Your child's name, age, and weight

* Any medical conditions your child has
* Any medicine your child is taking
* What your child swallowed—read the name off the container and spell it
* How much you think your child swallowed and when

If your child gets a chemical or other dangerous substance in his eyes: Flush them for at least ten minutes. The best way to do this? Place your child in the bathtub or shower (clothes and all if need be), and run tepid water directly into the eyes. Do this for ten full minutes despite his protests (and protest he will). Then call the doctor.

Important Information About Poisons and Vomiting

Syrup of ipecac is a drug that was used in the past to make children vomit after they had swallowed a poison. Although this may seem to make sense, making someone vomit is not a good poison treatment because having the poison travel back through the throat and mouth could actually cause more harm. Don't give your child syrup of ipecac or saltwater or do anything else to make him gag. If you have any syrup of ipecac at home, flush it down the toilet and throw away the container.

Source: The American Academy of Pediatrics (aap.org).

The Poison Hotline: 1-800-222-1222

If you suspect your child has eaten something poisonous (in little kids, that can range from a fistful of baby aspirins to cleaning liquids as well as real toxins) but he doesn't seem to be in real distress yet, call the poison control center at 1-800-222-1222. This is a nationwide toll-free number that will direct your call to a regional poison center, where a poison expert in your area is available twenty-four hours a day, seven days a week. (You can also call this number if you have a question about poisons or poison prevention.) Due to budget cuts, some states may be closing their regional offices. I recommend that you call to double-check that your region still has an active poison hotline before you need it.

TIP: If a permanent tooth is knocked out, time is extremely crucial. If your child is old enough, have him hold the tooth in the corner of his mouth or in the actual tooth socket and get to the dentist fast so that it can be saved. If you or your child is uncomfortable with this or if your child is too young, put the tooth in a glass of milk. Either way, get to the dentist as quickly as possible. Time is of the essence.

your babysitter (or your spouse) to refer to when you're not home. You should also give a copy to the teacher, coach, or nurse at your child's school, day-care program, or any kind of orga-

I Don't Think It's an Emergency, but Should I Call the Doctor?

Yes. If you are worried about something, trust your instincts and pick up the phone. There should be no attitude from your doctor if you jumped the gun when your daughter bit her lip badly. You should always feel free to call during office hours for everyday stuff and at any time for an emergency. Lots of times you may just need reassurance that what you're doing is right. Honestly, I'm far more concerned about parents who don't call me when they think something is wrong than about those who fret over calling unnecessarily. That's why I'm here!

TIP: If your child swallowed an object, like a Barbie shoe, for example (this happens), call your doctor and try to get an office appointment or see what your doctor recommends. Whether you end up at your doctor's office or an urgent care center, make sure to bring the other shoe so that the doctor can see the size and shape of the swallowed object. This also goes for things inserted into the nostril or ear.

nized sports or recreation program. If you go on vacation or a business trip without your children, leave a thorough medical file, including insurance information, with the caretaker, as well as a medical release form that allows that person to get care for your child. A medical release or consent form isn't necessary in a life-threatening emergency since paramedics and doctors are obligated to do whatever is necessary to try to save a person's life.

Assuming the illness or injury isn't life threatening, try to bring something to keep your child diverted while you're waiting, such as an mp3 player, handheld video games, crayons and paper, a deck of cards, or a book, favorite blankie, or cuddly toy. But if you left the house in a hurry, you may find yourself inventing some soothing stories or soft songs to comfort your child. If you have nothing—nada—ask the kindest-looking ED staffer for some unused tongue depressors and cotton balls that can become impromptu toys, or paper and pencil for drawing or tic-tac-toe.

One thing to leave home: **other small children,** if at all possible. They'll get in the way, get crabby, cause mayhem, and add a lot of stress. It's a good time to call in that favor from your neighbor.

A Product of Bad Breathing

"Breathing problems" are a common cause of unnecessary trips to the emergency department at three A.M. for kids who only have a tough case of the sniffles. Severe breathing difficulty is pretty easy to spot: Your child won't just be coughing and snuffling (which necessitates an office visit); she'll be having a hard time getting enough air. Her breathing might be either very fast (she's using the muscles in her neck and chest to breathe) or very shallow and slow (she's too tired to breathe adequately). If you're not sure if your child's breathing really constitutes an emergency, call your pediatrician. Go to the ED if you truly think it's urgent.

"He's Making a Whirring Sound"

Trying to describe your child's problem on the phone can be frustrating. Before you dial, do the following. It will save time.

- Be ready to give your child's stats, including name, age, gender, and medical history.
- Take your child's temperature just before you call. If the temp has risen or fallen during the last twenty-four hours or so, say so.

Got the Fever?

Parents are needlessly horrified by fevers. Remember, a high fever doesn't necessarily mean it's serious. Most severe infections that are accompanied by a high fever (such as meningitis and other bacterial blood infections) are less common now due to vaccinations. Fevers are the body's way of fighting infection, and kids tend to run higher fevers than adults. In many ways, it means the body is doing its job! What's more important is how your child *looks* and *responds to you*. If your child looks and acts sick or is extremely lethargic, call your pediatrician. Again, if you have a strong hunch that it's really an emergency, don't hesitate to go to the ED. When kids have a fever, it's okay to give Children's Tylenol (acetaminophen) or Children's Motrin (ibuprofen) if you think it will make them more comfortable. Just remember to tell the nurse and doctor about the fever reducer if you go to the ED. And *never give your child aspirin!* (See chapter 1 for more about aspirin.)

- If possible, have your child near the phone. That way you won't be running up and down stairs every time I ask you a question like "When was the last time your daughter threw up?"
- Make a list of any medications or treatments you've tried. And please remind us of any medical condition or special history

Dehydration . . . Why Does It Happen and What Does It Look Like?

Cases of dehydration are seen quite often, especially in children. Kids get dehydrated (run low on fluids) much quicker than adults because they have much smaller bodies. If they get a stomach bug or another infection that causes vomiting or diarrhea, dehydration can occur swiftly. If symptoms persist and fluid intake is not adequate, severe dehydration can be fatal.

Signs to watch out for: Listlessness, dry lips and mouth, crying without tears, or no urination over several hours (or very dark urine). Children suffering from dehydration often become so sick that they can't keep any food or water down. **Call your pediatrician pronto** if you spot any of the above symptoms. You may need to take your child to the ED to receive intravenous fluids. You can sometimes treat less severe cases of dehydration at home by giving a child a teaspoon of a pediatric oral rehydration fluid (such as Pedialyte) every five minutes or so. These mixtures contain a balance of fluid, sugar, and electrolytes and can be used to slowly rehydrate kids.

your child has—try as I might, it's very hard to remember every child's medical past.

- Have your pharmacy number handy in case a prescription needs to be called in.
- If you reach the doctor's service and leave your cell phone number, remember to leave your phone on! (And be sure it isn't stone dead or buried in the bottom of a briefcase or purse.)
- Have paper and pen handy to write down any instructions.
- Finally, try to relax. Kids get sick, they get injured, and—did I mention this?—they get sick. It's normal, but it can also be grueling and unsettling. Repeat to self: You will both get through this. Take a deep breath. There, that's better.

Drive or Take an Ambulance?

Obviously, if you fear your child's condition is very serious or could become life threatening (see page 172), call 911 and ask for an ambulance. Your child will receive potentially lifesaving treatment from the EMTs upon their arrival, and if your child's condition is *truly* life threatening, he will also get faster treatment at the ED.

In general, you *may* be able to drive to the ED if your child does not have a head, neck, or back injury, is awake and responding, is breathing without difficulty—and if you have another adult with you so one can comfort your child while the other drives. And, it should go without saying, you are sure you can drive (near) the speed limit, keep your wits about you, and not pass out behind the wheel. You don't need two emergencies.

Always talk to your pediatrician or another doctor before deciding to drive your child to the ED yourself. Sure, there may be rare circumstances in which you can't get an ambulance or can't reach your doctors (or perhaps anyone) by phone, in which case the closest functioning auto will have to suffice. But otherwise, get your pediatrician's opinion first.

One advantage of using your own car: You can drive to the hospital of your choice, meaning one you know is child friendly. When you call an ambulance, make sure you ask ahead of time if they'll take you to the hospital of your choice. If you don't request a specific hospital, they will typically go to the closest hospital—and as you know, the most convenient hospital may not be the best one for kids.

It's a Real Emergency ... Time to Take a Trip to the ED: The Six Commandments of Emergency Medical Care

1. Stay calm. If you freak out, so will your child.
2. If your child is unresponsive, call 911 and do the "ABC" check: A) Check the **A**irway to make sure it's not blocked. B) Check for **B**reathing—sounds of inhaled or exhaled air. C) Check for **C**irculation—your child's pulse. If you need to start CPR or do the Heimlich maneuver, the dispatcher can walk you through the steps while the paramedics are en route. Better yet, be prepared by taking a CPR class or take a refresher course.
3. Stop any bleeding by applying pressure on the wound. Remember to keep holding it (don't peek)! Every time you relieve the pressure, the bleeding will restart. So hold on and apply pressure for at least ten minutes. (Be prepared: Scalp and tongue wounds are especially bloody, so try not to overreact. Follow the same steps for these wounds.)
4. Don't move your child if you suspect a head, neck, or back injury. With any serious head injury, assume your child also has a broken neck, just in case. Cover your child with a blanket and wait for the paramedics.
5. If a finger or toe has been cut off (gruesome, but it happens), apply pressure to the wound, then place a cloth, towel, or

plastic bag around the body part and ice it. Make sure it isn't directly touching the ice and is protected. The body part can probably be reattached if the surgery's done within six hours.

6. On the chance that your child will need emergency surgery, don't give him or her anything to eat or drink. It's much safer to get anesthesia on an empty stomach.

If Only All Parents Were Like You ...

When you get to the ED, you will undoubtedly meet many parents who are not prudent, not reasonable, and *definitely* not smart parents. They've brought their child to the ED for something nonserious that could have waited for an office visit. For a variety of reasons, families rely on the ED for everyday health care. Sometimes, it's because they don't have a primary care doctor or health insurance. Others simply abuse the ED by using it as a walk-in clinic for convenience. But emergency care won't keep a child healthy; it isn't comprehensive care from a pediatrician who knows your child's medical history and any chronic conditions, something an emergency physician can't possibly offer.

Other parents in the ED will have children who are genuinely sick and in danger—but all that could have been prevented by a simple call to their pediatrician or trip to a free clinic days before, when their toddler's symptoms (such as a bad earache) first became worrisome. Most EDs in America are unnecessarily clogged with crying kids who have fevers, ear infections, red faces and lips (from a coughing or choking fit), and pinkeye, and other little ones who could be home cuddling the family pet if their parents had simply acted earlier or called the pediatrician and *accurately described* their symptoms.

Whatever brought them there, all of these parents have two things in common: They're contributing to overcrowding and preventing people who are experiencing true emergencies—maybe your child—from getting prompt care.

Suspicious Minds

If you find yourself a frequent visitor to your local hospital's ED, expect to get scrutinized rather heavily if your child is accident prone and his or her file is thicker than the Yellow Pages. If you come in with a child who looks like a raccoon with two black eyes from walking into a door, you will get asked some tough questions about what happened. Be prepared to answer them honestly and without attitude.

The medical staff is obligated to ask questions about any child who comes in with bruises, eye injuries, or any damage that could possibly be from the hands of an abusive parent or care worker. It's estimated that 10 percent of children brought to the ED with traumatic injuries are victims of child abuse, so don't take offense. The hospital staff is just doing its job. If they even suspect the possibility of physical abuse, they are required to notify local authorities. You could even get a visit from a social worker who is doing a "well-being check" to make sure the child is safe and in a good home environment.

A tip: Sometimes scars, discolorations due to a skin condition, or even certain kinds of birthmarks will arouse the hospital staff's suspicion. For example, Asian and African-American children often have blue and black birthmarks on their backs that can resemble bruising. It's a good idea to have all such marks documented with your pediatrician so that you don't have any difficulty proving your innocence to (thankfully) conscientious nurses, social workers, or other medical or children's welfare workers.

What to Say—and Not Say— About P-A-I-N

It's a bad idea to fib about or downplay the possibility of pain to your child when unpleasant tests or procedures need to be done. After all, you wouldn't be in the ED if there wasn't something really wrong. Kids are pretty smart creatures. You know your kid best, of course, but you shouldn't try to trick your child into thinking that getting his or her arm reset, for example, isn't going to hurt.

If your child needs a painful procedure, it's best to be honest and tell him that it will hurt for a moment but then everything will be okay. Of course, that may not be completely honest, but it's honest enough. Don't lie and say it won't hurt to assuage his fear or give him hope. That will only work once, plus then he'll be certain that every subsequent procedure will be agonizing, no matter what you say.

Young kids will be helped by a simple explanation of what is going to happen and maybe even a drawing, while older kids may appreciate more information. Making comparisons to other ouches can be helpful; for example, if your child is afraid of a shot, you can say it will hurt for a second, just like a pinch or a bug bite, but then it'll stop. The pediatrician may ask him to yell "Ouch!" or use another tactic to distract him from the pain.

Do your best to get him some real pain relief whenever possible, too. If your child needs to have a shot, blood drawn, or stitches, ask about "ouchless" options. For example, there's a numbing cream the doctor can apply to his skin, but it takes about one hour to work. For minor lacerations, you can ask the doctor if skin tape (called Steri-Strips) or skin glue might work instead of stitches.

The Waiting Game

Even if the pediatric area looks cheery, the emergency department isn't the most pleasant place. It's often crowded, chaotic, and full of anxious, sick people. Of course, how bad it is depends on the time of day (four to eight P.M. is worst), the day of the week (weekends and Mondays are terrible), whether it's a holiday, how many people are there, and what kind of shape they're in.

Unfortunately, as mentioned, because a lot of people don't have insurance or primary care doctors these days, the ED is often filled with people who should be in a doctor's office. Emergency departments must treat everyone, despite their ability to pay, so that means the place can be crowded. You'll see people with bad colds and flu as well as broken bones or worse. Expect a long wait. And don't be fooled if the waiting room looks nearly empty; it could be that every spot in the treatment area is full or that much of the staff is in one room trying to save a person's life.

Be your child's advocate, and feel free to express any concerns. If your child is in a lot of pain, say so. If you feel the care your child is getting isn't up to snuff, tell the doctor or nurse in a respectful manner. But talk yourself down if you get impatient or irritated. It just won't help. It may even be a good idea to show a little love to the staff and thank them as they go about their work. Getting hostile or demanding isn't going to win you any brownie points. It shouldn't affect your child's care if you really get belligerent or go off on some poor, tired staffer—but it could.

Just remember, the nurses and doctors are likely doing the best they can, usually under very trying circumstances. You've seen the TV versions, so you have a bit of an idea what's happening. Your stress level is probably off the charts, but don't take it out on the staffers. Your child may be one of ten patients they're seeing at one time, any or all of whom could require more urgent care because they are severely ill while your child's life isn't in danger.

Fast-Tracking in the ED?

Can you really get through the emergency department swiftly by schmoozing the front-desk nurse or sweet-talking the triage nurse? Well, let's see . . . did you happen to bring a hot pizza or some gourmet chocolates along with you? Great, but that still may not help much. It might bump you in front of the woman with the sprained ankle, but the ED staffers won't let two people have a heart attack just because you brought goodies.

The best way to speed things along is, again, to **call your pediatrician first** so your pediatrician can call the ED and let them know you're coming. If your doctor talks to the ED doctor, there's a good chance that will get you seen faster, especially if the problem is serious or the two docs know each other and often help each other out.

The second way to speed things along is to be nice. Assertive, but nice.

If you find yourself waiting a really long time (let's say over an hour), it's okay to ask the desk person for an update and find out where your child is on the list. Then pile on some praise: "Boy, I see how busy you are." ("And those scrubs you're wearing are fetching." Just kidding about that part.)

When the clock hands have gone around again and you need to notch up the nudging, say, "My daughter over there is just miserable. I'd appreciate any update you can give us." If you're nice about it and keep your voice down (you don't want the others in the waiting room to know you're working it a bit), you might just climb a spot or two ahead of the patients sitting beside you—if their situations aren't more medically serious, that is.

As for the wait . . . as ED docs like to say, "We're not sleeping back there." Well, maybe one is, in the back closet. But she's been in the ED for twenty-one hours.

Tips from the Trenches

Want insights from an ED insider? Listen to someone who's spent more than ten years handling emergencies in several types of EDs: my old friend Karin Berger-Sadow, MD. She's currently medical director of PM Pediatrics, an urgent care center in Mamaroneck, New York, and she's also the former director of the pediatric emergency department at Mt. Sinai Hospital in New York City. Here are her most important emergency tips:

1. Don't give your child anything to eat or drink if there is a possibility that your child may need sedation or anesthesia for a surgical procedure. This bears repeating. We see children who need immediate surgery, but we can't sedate them because the parent gave them food in the waiting room or on the ride over. Bad idea! So if you think there's a chance your child will need anesthesia or sedation in order to treat an injury or illness—such as surgery to treat abdominal pain or a procedure to realign a broken bone—don't give her anything to eat or drink on your way to the ED or while you're waiting in the ED.

2. Say what you *see*, not what you read. Patients will say, "My daughter's lethargic and has labored breathing," because they just read those terms when looking up conditions on the Internet. That tells the ED doctor nothing. If a doctor says, "The child is lethargic and has labored breathing," it means she's semi-unconscious and likely needs to go on a ventilator immediately. When a parent says it, it means she's sniffling and watching TV instead of running around.

"Respiratory distress" is another term to avoid. About ten parents a day say their child has respiratory distress. Thankfully, we see only one child a week who really does, and that child usually needs to have a breathing tube inserted. So say what you see. Is she limping? Is she cringing in pain after coughing? Nodding off at the dinner table? Say that—don't use medical terminology.

3. Say the magic words. If your child's symptoms have worsened while you've been waiting to be seen, tell the triage nurse, "My child's getting worse." Then describe what's changed. You won't be able to snow the triage nurse if it isn't true, but if it is, it will get his or her attention. It means what was written down on the form three hours ago may not be valid now.

4. If necessary, ask for a "doctor-to-doctor" call. If you've been waiting an excessive period of time (over an hour), you really believe your child needs to be seen immediately or his condition is getting worse, and you cannot get the triage nurse to notice you, call your pediatrician and ask her to call the ED again. Ask your pediatrician to speak directly to one of the ED docs to let them know you're waiting to be seen.

Should I Stay or Should I Go?

In general, you should always try to stick by your child's side throughout testing and treatment. For most parents, this is the only choice they'd consider anyway. What's more, studies have shown that, providing parents aren't disruptive, having a parent present during a trauma can comfort the child and help the medical team if they have questions that need immediate answers. Your child will be less frightened, so will you, and it'll make things easier for the ED staff. (For example, if the doctor orders an MRI or X-ray, you can ease your child's anxiety over the scary-looking equipment.)

Staying with your child also allows you to **make sure the correct procedure is being done.** A hospital accredited by The Joint Commission is required to get two patient identifiers (like name and birth date) every time staff members draw blood or take your child away for a test, and being there to confirm that information is the sign of a smart parent who stays smart even when under pressure.

The Meltdown Factor

There's a big exception to the above, however. And that big exception is, of course, parents who become hysterical. A pediatric emergency department is not the place for the squeamish or highly excitable. In fact, when I did my residency at the Mt. Sinai pediatric emergency department in New York City, I learned one thing pretty fast: Pediatric emergency doctors often get two patients at once—the child and the parent. I had a reminder of this recently. While I was treating a nine-year-old girl for an allergic reaction, her mom had a panic attack. Then the mom became the patient. Then the little girl freaked out about her mom, on top of having an allergic reaction. It brought back memories.

Most parents are usually fine—until you have to insert an IV, do a spinal tap, intubate their baby, or put their frantic child in soft restraints in order to do stitches or other delicate procedures. In my experience, even the coolest cats tend to freak out over these four common necessities. Pediatric ED docs are usually adept at calming down parents, although sometimes they do have to ask one to exit the treatment area for the benefit of the child. And everyone else. However, most moms and dads know when they need to get some fresh air or take a strategic bathroom break. If you think you cannot remain calm during a particular procedure, tell the nurse or doctor. They've been through this before. In fact, probably eighteen minutes ago.

Dire Situations

If your child's situation is life threatening, some hospitals will let you decide if you want to be present during drastic treatment measures, such as when a child is being resuscitated or undergoing an invasive procedure to save his or her life. However, many hospitals have no written guidelines for these situations, so simply ask. It may be important; parents who have lost children in the ED say they believe being there benefited their child and helped with their own grieving.

Do You Need a Plastic Surgeon?

Let's say your child has a nasty cut that seems like it may leave a scar in a visible place. Should you get a plastic surgeon to tend to it? Go to the emergency department? Or have your pediatrician close the wound in an office visit?

It depends on the location and how deep the cut is. If possible, talk to your pediatrician before heading to the ED. Sometimes smaller lacerations can be treated and closed with new super skin glues or Steri-Strips right in your doctor's office. If the injury warrants a trip to the emergency department, the ED docs stitch people up all the time, so they are pretty expert at making fine cross-stitches and being sensitive to scarring issues. However, if a laceration is very jagged, many layers deep, or located over a joint, or there is potential for nerve damage, then I would recommend having a plastic surgeon do the job. I'd also recommend seeing a plastic surgeon for large lacerations on the face, mainly for cosmetic reasons.

Have an Exit Plan

The initial crisis is over and your child either has been treated and is about to be released or is being admitted to the hospital. If your child is being released, there's just one little thing you're waiting on: your discharge paperwork. It will include instructions on how to care for the illness or injury at home, any follow-up treatment that may be necessary from your regular doctor, and a number to call if you have problems or complications. Some EDs will send a record of your visit directly to your pediatrician; ask about this.

It is really important that you call your pediatrician when you get home and explain everything that happened. Why is this vital? So your pediatrician can document the ED visit in your child's medical records and follow up on any concerns or new developments. For example, if your child was treated for a severe allergic reaction, your doctor needs to figure out what caused the problem and how to avoid it in the future.

Hug It Out

Kids can be pretty traumatized by a trip to the ED, so when you get home, talk about what happened and reassure your child. Answer any questions that may come up. Sometimes, younger children work out their feelings through play, by drawing pictures, or by talking about the hospital. Experts say this is a normal way for them to "desensitize" themselves. If they got a shot or had blood taken, they might want to play with a toy medical kit and pretend to be a nurse giving shots. Reliving the experience can be their way of dealing with their feelings once the emergency is over.

CHAPTER 5 POP QUIZ ANSWER KEY

1. How do you find the best ED or urgent care facility for your child? The answer is C: Check out your options before an emergency strikes and select one that is Joint Commission accredited, or in a Joint Commission–accredited hospital, and equipped to treat children. (Page 167.)

2. How do you know if it's really an emergency? The answer is C—your gut tells you this is the real deal, so get help fast. (Page 171.)

3. When is it okay to drive to the ED? The answers are B and D—when your child does not have a head, neck, or back injury, is awake and responding, is breathing without problems, *and* if two adults are in a car that has plenty of gas. (Page 182.)

4. What's the secret for getting fast service in the ED? The answer is D. Being super-nice to the staff *and* asking your pediatrician to call ahead may help. (Page 188.)

5. How do you find out if you local hospital's ED is kid friendly? The answer is B. Talk to your doctor, do some homework, and check out the hospital's status on www.qualitycheck.org. (Page 167.)

6. What should you do if your toddler swallows a pink Barbie shoe? The answers are A and D. Call the doctor; then, regardless of whether you go to the office or the ED, bring the mate to that shoe so that the doctor can see its size and shape. (Page 178.)

7. Should you stay with your child in the ED, even when he goes for tests? The simple answer is D, or yes. But really, how can you even ask? (Page 190.)

8. Will your kids ever grow up and stop having accidents and getting sick in the middle of the night? The answers are A, B, C, and D. It's called being a parent. Your job never stops.

Chapter 6

If Your Child Has to Be Hospitalized, Where Should You Go?

Choosing the Best Hospital for a Kid Does Not Involve a Dart and a Map

POP QUIZ

Do you know where the best hospital is for your child? Do you know how to get there? And are you *sure* it's the best? Take this quiz and find out. Answers can be found at the end of the chapter. (Tip: There may be more than one correct answer.) If you get all seven questions right, feel free to skip to the next chapter. Otherwise, read on and try to absorb this chapter like a sponge. It could save your child's life one day. Even tomorrow . . .

1. If you live in the U.S, the odds that your child will be hospitalized this year are . . .
    A. 1 in 5, more or less
    B. 1 in 25, more or less
    C. 1 in 83, precisely
    D. 1 in 5,000, according to government supercomputers

2. Before you check your child (or anyone else) into a hospital, you should make sure it's accredited by . . .
    A. *Consumer Reports* magazine
    B. Your local Better Business Bureau

   C. Someone you know who's been a patient there
   D. The Joint Commission
   E. All of the above

3. Which statement best describes teaching hospitals?
   A. They're public hospitals funded by the government for use by schoolteachers at every level, from preschool through college.
   B. They're facilities that typically provide excellent care and are often part of world-leading institutions, but that also teach new doctors.
   C. They're hospitals affiliated with universities in which university students and faculty receive free care, as long as they agree to undergo experimental treatments and participate in clinical studies.
   D. This is a medical slang term for hospitals that teach other hospitals what *not* to do.

4. Which of the following is the name of an anti-abduction system used in many hospitals?
   A. HUGS
   B. KIDLOK
   C. The Parent Retinal ID system
   D. The Every Child Left Inside program

5. What is a common visual tool that good hospitals use to help children communicate their pain level?
   A. The "How Much Can Elmo Stand?" Rating Scale
   B. Photographs ranging from an arm being bitten by a mosquito to fingers being slammed in a drawer
   C. The Wong-Baker FACES Pain Rating Scale
   D. The Army Field Manual's Universal Hand Gestures

6. Which question should you ask before selecting a hospital to perform surgery on your child?
   A. What is your hospital's volume-and-success rate for the particular procedure my child needs?

B. Is the surgeon a specialist in pediatric surgery?

C. Do you have an on-staff pediatric anesthesiologist?

D. All of the above

7. Which practice has been found to reduce the number of medication errors in hospitals by two-thirds?

    A. Having a pharmacist participate in daily rounds

    B. Asking two nurses to be present whenever medication is given

    C. Posting a notice of the child's medications in red ink next to the child's bed

    D. Requesting that a doctor personally administer all medication

As a smart parent, you probably do everything possible to keep your children safe, healthy, and happy. That means: Seat belts. Bike helmets. Nutritious meals. Plenty of sleep. Lots of TLC. Only educational TV. That's your job, 24/7/365—at least until they're eighteen or so. As a mom, my children are my number one priority (my hubby is up there, too!). However, kids get sick or injured, despite parents' best efforts, and sometimes need to be admitted to the hospital. Much as you hate the idea, your kid(s) will probably join these ranks at some point. But don't let that throw you. Instead, be as prepared as you can be. While a hospital experience will be extremely stressful for both you and your child, it will be more so if you have to start from scratch in the ambulance.

Every minute of every day, children are admitted to hospitals for dozens of reasons—for tests, to set a broken leg, to correct a hernia, to treat a chronic condition, and much more. Regardless of why your child might need a hospital stay, two things are musts: You *must* choose the absolute best hospital for your child, and you *must* have a solid game plan.

I'm here to help you. In this chapter, we're going to deal with the first must, which is *finding the best hospital for your child*. In chapter 7, we'll deal with the other must: having a game plan to see your child through a hospital stay.

If It's Not Accredited, Keep Searching

Always, always check to see if a hospital is accredited by The Joint Commission, or "The Joint," as it's affectionately called by the folks who work there. The mission of this good group is to help hospitals (and other health care organizations) provide the safest and best health care possible. You might not have heard of The Joint Commission, but you can bet doctors, nurses, hospitals, and everyone else in health care has. That's because it delivers what amounts to a report card on hospitals. Bad report card, big trouble. Good report card—which means meeting extremely high standards and safety goals—and the hospital earns The Joint Commission's Gold Seal of Approval.

So how do you find out if a hospital is accredited? Just go to www.qualitycheck.org. Hospitals voluntarily seek accreditation, and then The Joint Commission makes unannounced inspections (called surveys) to review the hospital's medical and nursing care, infection prevention and control procedures, facility safety, medication management, and other health and safety standards. Frankly, if The Joint Commission hasn't checked out a hospital, I wouldn't check in.

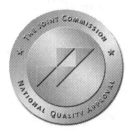

Look for The Joint Commission's Gold Seal of Approval on hospital websites and brochures.

What Are the Odds?

More than three million children are hospitalized in the United States every year. Since there are about seventy-five million kids aged seventeen and under, statistically **your child has a 1 in 25 chance of being admitted to a hospital this year.** Okay, that's not technically true. Your child's individual odds could be much higher or lower, depending on geographic location, age, after-school activities, and dozens of other niggling variables. So let's hope your odds of joining this group are much smaller. But let's say 1 in 25, just to emphasize that, yes, it can happen to your kid.

How a Doctor (aka Dr. Jen) Chooses a Hospital

So far, I've been pretty lucky. None of my kids has ever spent a night in a hospital except when they were born, and they pretty much slept through that. But I've logged thousands of hours in hospital pediatric departments. And—gulp—I know that my chance to be an anxious mom who's admitting her child and dealing with all the issues and worries that brings will come. After all, my husband and I do have three kids, so the odds almost guarantee it. I just hope my kids are in their late seventies when it happens!

When my turn to be worried-mom-with-kid-in-hospital arrives, I'll have a powerful advantage, and it's not my hospital parking lot pass. I've had the privilege of guiding thousands of parents and children through the hospital process. From these

experiences—which run the gamut from miraculous to nightmar-
ish (although most are beautifully brief and uneventful)—I've
learned invaluable strategies about choosing the best hospital
and getting through the journey as safely as possible. I know exactly what I would do as a mom for my own children. Not that
I wouldn't be a nervous wreck every step of the way. A mom's a
mom. (I'm not leaving out dads here. I know they worry too, but
they don't always admit or show it.)

So, how does a pediatrician/mom pick the best hospital
for her own child? Or find out about the pediatric specialists
there? Or check out the quality of the pediatric medical equipment? And find out how well they treat pain? Or discover
whether the hospital's shift changes—an especially risky time
in a pediatric ward—are run like the changing of the guard
at Buckingham Palace or more like the Keystone Cops are in
charge?

I have great access to information. I know which children's
hospitals kick butt for specific treatments and which are merely
great PR machines. I can phone colleagues who've done stints
at most every notable pediatric center in the U.S. and several
abroad. But *you can get this inside information, too*! It just takes
some sleuthing. I'm going to show you how to do that and give
you insider tips to make it easier, so you can pick a hospital as
well as I can.

Shouldn't I Just Go to
My Pediatrician's Hospital?

No. At least not without checking it out first. With luck, you'll
find that the hospital where your pediatrician has privileges
is, indeed, the best choice for your child. But it may not be.
You remember from chapter 5 that in an emergency, the closest hospital—the one where the paramedics want to take your

child—could be your worst option. The hospital your child desperately needs might be miles farther away, and the failure to go straight there could prove a problem. But remember, if time is of the essence, any hospital may have to suffice.

But we're going to talk about situations in which you *do* have a little more time—whether it's six days or six months—to decide which hospital would be a perfect fit for what your child needs to have done.

For example, does your child need a specialist in orthopedics, asthma, or epilepsy? Or kidney transplants or cancer treatments? Many hospitals specialize in certain conditions or diseases. They're not one-size-fits-all. The pediatric expert in respiratory conditions who would be perfect for your kid might work in a children's hospital that's two hours away.

I know too many parents who think, "Look, if it were really serious, I'd just take my son to ABC Hospital, which is the most prominent in the area and has a national reputation." That can be flawed thinking. The grand old hospital that everyone in town reveres may indeed be a nationally acclaimed center of excellence for, say, breast cancer or heart surgery. But that doesn't mean it's outstanding for the treatment your child needs. It might just be decent for that. The grand old hospital is not going to tell you this, of course. **The only way to find out is to do your own research.** So it's time to investigate.

Start with Your Doc, and Keep Your Priorities Straight

As with finding a doctor, your first step in finding the right hospital is to create a list of your options. Start by picking your pediatrician's brain. Ask about the pluses and minuses of the hospital(s) where he or she has privileges, and also whether there are others your pediatrician would recommend for the problem your child's facing. Once you've got a list, these are your five determining factors, in this order:

1. Which hospitals are accredited by The Joint Commission
2. What procedures or treatments your child needs
3. Which hospitals are covered by your health insurance
4. Which hospital(s) your pediatrician has privileges in
5. Which are conveniently located

Why isn't insurance coverage the top priority? In the end, it may be the deciding factor for the majority of us. (Those of us with health insurance are lucky to even have it.) But getting the best possible care is *always* the goal, and if the excellent hospital that your child really needs for lifesaving surgery or a highly specific treatment is outside your health insurance carrier's network, you need to find that out. Ultimately, you may not be able to use the best hospital, but you can ask the doctors in your hospital to consult with the doctors in your first-choice hospital, or you can see them independently for a second opinion (which may or may not be covered by your insurance plan).

Now that you've got a ranked list, ask your doc some follow-up questions: Do any of these hospitals have affiliations with other well-known hospitals? (A good sign.) Which one does your doc think is the absolute best at treating the problem your child has? Are there any hospitals much farther away that might be even better? Should you consider one of them? Which hospital would your doctor choose in your situation? Only then, after talking to your pediatrician, are you ready to call your health insurer and find out which hospitals are covered.

What's Routine? What's Specialized?

If you ask doctors which hospital they would choose for their own kids, most would say a children's hospital or teaching hospital for specialized care, but for "routine stuff" (and the definition of "routine" can vary from doc to doc), they'd likely go to their local community hospital.

I basically agree with this strategy. But how do you decide if the care your child needs is routine or specialized? And really, is anything routine when it comes to *your* kid?

Your pediatrician can fill you in on what he or she considers to be "routine." For example, any competent hospital's emergency department can treat a serious ear infection or set a broken arm. (That's assuming the hospital is accredited by The Joint Commission.) However, if your child needs major surgery or is being treated for something that's complex, rare, or mysterious, it may be worth the travel challenges to choose the more specialized but more distant hospital. If it's really too far, maybe you can go there once, spend a day developing a treatment plan, and then get a referral to a doctor/hospital closer to home. Your goal—I don't have to tell you—is to get the best doctor and hospital to help your child.

Teaching Hospitals, Community Hospitals, Children's Hospitals: What's the Diff?

A **teaching hospital** not only delivers medical care to patients, but it also provides clinical education and training to future and current doctors, nurses, and other health professionals. Some teaching hospitals also do research and are centers for experimental, innovative, and technically sophisticated services. Teaching hospitals are generally affiliated with a school of medicine, and some may even be owned by a university or be part of an entire health system or network.

Traditional or **community hospitals** treat patients of all ages. **Children's hospitals** only treat kids, although they often also do research on childhood diseases. Both types of hospitals can also be teaching hospitals or affiliated with teaching hospitals, so ask about those relationships and any "what if" scenarios you might be wondering about.

Should I Choose a Children's Hospital?

Smart question. One big advantage of children's hospitals is that they are totally tuned into young patients. That's all they do and see, and so their approach is through the eyes of a child. The physicians, surgeons, anesthesiologists, residents, pharmacists, and nurses are specially trained and deeply knowledgeable about childhood illnesses, proper doses for little ones, pediatric-sized equipment, and treating young bodies. The staff also understands the emotional issues that young patients and their families go through and knows ways to minimize the anxiety. Many children's hospitals see children with rare illnesses into adulthood, allowing for steady, continuous care.

Children's hospitals often serve as the pediatric training ground for medical schools, so you and your child benefit not only from the hospital's highly trained clinicians and instructors but also from the many medical students and residents. Even though they're still learning their craft, young docs are also up on the latest research, education, and technology. They're closely supervised by pediatric fellows and attending specialists (see page 232 to learn more about the types of doctors working in hospitals), so you don't have to worry about anyone flying solo. Personally, I like the idea of young, eager, brainiac students trying to outdo themselves to impress their teachers (your child's doctors) *and* you and your child (the patient).

The kid focus at pediatric hospitals is usually reflected in the atmosphere. Many pride themselves on having a whimsical, cheery décor. You might see aquariums, skylights, toys, games, computers—all designed to be a distraction from the rigors of being hospitalized. Actually, all hospitals try to make their pediatric wings fun and kid friendly, but in children's hospitals, the whole place is like that.

However, here's what's most important: Studies show that even "routine" procedures at children's hospitals are generally safer and have fewer complications and lower mortality rates than those done on kids in adult hospital settings.

Don't Get Me Wrong: Community Hospitals Can Kick Butt

Having said all of the above, don't misunderstand me. I'm not downplaying the importance and high quality of many, many local hospitals. Many are superb. I know a lot of extremely talented doctors who work in community hospitals, including a few who would not hesitate to egg my house in the middle of the night if they thought I was insinuating that their institutions provide anything less than top-flight care. Your neighborhood hospital may be perfect for your child's needs, especially for "routine" stuff done under your pediatrician's eye. Talk to your doctor about all these issues, and make a plan together. Whatever hospital you choose, your aim remains the same: Make sure the doctor and staff come highly recommended and offer quality, safe care.

Great Websites for Checking Out Hospitals

In addition to The Joint Commission's website www.quality check.org, mentioned earlier in this chapter, these sites tell you how hospitals rate in patient care, safety, and other vital areas. So put the kids to bed, grab a mug of your favorite tea, and settle in with your computer—*now*, when no one's sick and there's no emergency. Smart parents are like Boy Scouts: always prepared.

www.childrenshospitals.net
If you need a children's hospital—there are about 250 in the U.S.—go to this site and use their "Find a Children's Hospital" search. You can search by geography, programs, services, research topics, and more, all courtesy of the National Association of Children's Hospitals and Related Institutions.

www.leapfroggroup.org
The Leapfrog Group is a nonprofit organization made up of large companies and other entities that buy health care for their employees. It ranks how well many health care providers (including hospitals) meet standards of quality and safety. This is a good site to find hospitals, and its "Compare Hospitals Now" option can be particularly helpful. It also gives all hospitals what it calls a Safe Practices Score: a rating according to how many of twenty-seven measures the hospital has taken to prevent medical mistakes.

www.hospitalcompare.hhs.gov
Most hospital comparisons focus more on adult care (prostate cancer, heart bypass) than children's ailments. Luckily, this government site offers information on pediatric treatments and allows you to compare quality, patient satisfaction, and pricing. (You can also find information on newborn care, such as neonatal intensive care units.) Of particular use to many parents is info comparing the quality of asthma care in many hospitals.

health.usnews.com/directories/hospital-directory/
The American Hospital Association and *U.S. News and World Report* magazine have linked up to provide a directory of five thousand hospitals. Its search mechanism is handy for finding the types of services a hospital provides, its accreditation, the number of full-time registered nurses there, its family support services, its admissions, etc.

Time to Chat with the Hospital Rep

Okay, you have your list of contenders. Now you need to go straight to the source. First, check out each hospital's website. A lot of the questions below can be answered there. But I'd also call the hospital's admissions office and ask at least the first six questions if I were considering using that hospital for *any reason*—removing my husband's gall bladder, replacing my eighty-year-old aunt's hip, or getting ear tubes for my kid.

1. **What percentage of the staff physicians are board certified?** About 85 percent of all U.S. physicians are board certified. The percentage of certified physicians may be even higher at a large urban hospital. "Board certified" means that a doctor has passed an exam given by a specialty board of the American Board of Medical Specialties in one or more of twenty-four areas.

2. **May I see your recent patient-satisfaction survey results?** If the hospital is doing a good job, they should want to share that. If the results aren't up to snuff, it's better to find out now.

3. **What percentage of the nurses are RNs?** Registered nurses have more training than licensed practical nurses (LPNs). On average, about 85 percent of a hospital's nursing staff are RNs.

4. **Does a pharmacist participate in daily rounds, at least in the intensive care unit?** You want the answer to be yes. A study found such participation reduced medication mistakes by two-thirds.

5. **What other hospitals are you affiliated with?** Good to know, right?

6. **Do you have a written description of your services and fees?** If yes, ask them to e-mail you a copy of it.

7. **May I tour the pediatric floor?** If it's a children's hospital, ask to see the specific section where your child will be. For

more info on exactly what you need to learn during this tour, see page 212.

8. **Do you have pediatric-sized supplies and equipment?** For example, ask about kid-sized beds, oxygen masks, resuscitation kits, and IV kits. See page 167 in chapter 5 for more info on this necessity.

9. **Does your hospital have a pediatric intensive care unit?** If not, do you have an arrangement with a nearby hospital that does?

10. **Does your pediatric department have staff available around the clock that is trained in pediatric emergencies?**

11. **Do you have a fall-prevention program?** Why is this so important? One study found a hospital fall rate of 33 percent for pediatric patients, more than double that for adults. A fall-prevention program means the hospital has age-appropriate devices—such as side rails on child-sized beds and bubble-top cribs for toddlers to keep kids from falling out of bed—as well as systems to keep them from slipping on wet floors and tripping over equipment. Most falls involve kids under two years old rolling out of bed or falling while walking.

12. **What programs do you have to ensure the security of pediatric patients?** One baby abducted from the nursery is one too many. (A custody battle increases the need to make sure your child is safe.) My hospital uses an electronic monitor bracelet system called HUGS. If an infant is moved anywhere outside the designated newborn area, a loud buzzer sounds and the doors lock. This can be very disconcerting, but in a good way. Most hospitals use similar monitoring devices in their nurseries, but not all hospitals use these on their general pediatric floor. Make sure to ask what abduction-prevention system your hospital uses on the pediatric floor.

13. **To help children communicate their pain, do you use the Wong-Baker FACES Pain Rating Scale or another visual**

tool? Ask this even if your child is an infant. A hospital that doesn't isn't adept at working with children.

14. **Do you have any child life specialists?** These professionals make sure kids in the hospital understand what's going on. They help them feel more comfortable and use teaching tools to reduce stress. (See more on the role of the child life specialist on page 212.) Social workers can also fill this role, but be sure they have experience with pediatric patients.

15. **What are the rules for visitors? May parents stay overnight with their kids, and what are the accommodations?** The hospital's admissions rep can give you this info, but re-ask the question during your tour of the pediatric floor. The accommodations may not be plush, by the way, but the important thing is that you can be with your child.

If your child is having surgery, add these questions.

16. **What is your hospital's volume and success rate for the particular procedure my child needs?** So ask, "How many surgeries like my child's do you do weekly, monthly, or annually, and how many of those are successful?" You *must* get this info; it's vital. The more surgeries of the type your child needs that a hospital does, the more likely the outcome will be successful. (Practice does make perfect.) The hospital should readily tell you how often the procedure is done there, how often the surgeon does it, and how well the patients fare. (You should also be able to find much of this info on the websites given in this chapter.)

17. **Is the surgeon a specialist in pediatric surgery?** (Remember: Kids are different from adults!)

18. **Do you have an on-staff pediatric anesthesiologist?** This is a must. An anesthesiologist who isn't a pediatric specialist shouldn't be handling children's surgeries.

What on Earth Is a Child Life Specialist?

These are professionals trained in pediatric health care who work with parents and kids (including siblings) to lower everyone's stress and increase their understanding of what's going on. Child life specialists can be particularly helpful during a difficult or unexpected illness, after the death of a loved one, or after violent acts or natural disasters. They focus on psychosocial issues and offer effective coping strategies for young patients and their families. Sometimes, this involves teaching children relaxation methods so they can calm themselves during a difficult procedure or letting kids play with real or pretend medical equipment so they know what will happen during a test or treatment—fear of the unknown can be the scariest part. Their efforts often reduce the need for sometimes risky sedatives and pain medications.

It's Tour Time!

If at all possible, take a tour of the hospital's pediatric department—especially the area your child will be in—before sending your child there. This is often the tiebreaker between two hospitals that seem equally qualified. When the elevator doors open, here's exactly what to look for and what to ask the person who's showing you around. By the way, I'd also re-ask your tour guide any questions from the list on pages 209 through 211 that you want more details on.

- Does the area look squeaky clean? And smell that way, too?
- Is the pediatric floor colorful and appealing? Do posters, books, toys, video games, DVDs, and other amusements abound? Such trappings are not only an indication that your child will be less anxious there but also that the staff handles children exclusively.
- Is there a specific treatment room that's a safe haven from germs—meaning a place where procedures and all IV insertions are performed? There should be, and there should also be signs announcing the room's sacred use, so no one is tempted to eat a pizza in there.
- Are there signs on doors indicating which children require respiratory isolation, contact isolation, or just plain isolation; what protective gear must be worn upon entering; and any other precautions that must be taken? Are masks or gowns accessible right outside those doors? Is *everyone* following those precautions? If you don't see any caution signs, ask why. I wouldn't admit my child to a pediatric floor that wasn't handling delicate cases on a daily basis.
- Do doctors, nurses, and all other staffers wash their hands every time they enter a child's room? Hand washing is a *must,* so particularly keep an eye out for this. But also try to notice if they clean stethoscopes between patients.
- Ask to see the Wong-Baker FACES Pain Rating Scale they use to help children indicate their pain level.
- Do they indeed have child-sized beds and other mini-equipment? You were told "yes" on the phone, but confirm that with your own eyes. If you're not sure, ask your guide to point out the kiddie-sized apparatus.
- Does the hospital provide child-sized pajamas and robes, or is it okay to bring your child's own PJs? If the kids are in adult-sized gowns, that's a bad sign.
- Ask for a sample menu and eyeball the food being served. Does the food look appealing to kids? Would you eat it?

Need to Find a Hospital Abroad?

If your family is visiting or moving to a foreign country, I urge you to plan ahead. (Gee, surprised by that? That's pretty much me in a nutshell—be prepared and plan ahead.) You need to be sure that you'll have good hospitals at your disposal. Luckily, finding this out couldn't be easier. Joint Commission International accredits health care organizations in dozens of countries. Go to www.jointcommissioninternational.org, click on "JCI-Accredited Organizations," and you'll see a listing of hospitals that you can trust to have good health and safety standards. Before you leave, print out the accredited hospitals in the country(ies) you're visiting so you have that information handy. Just in case.

- Ask to see the children's playroom. Is it clean? Fun? Ask your guide how often they clean the toys and how they control the risk of infection.
- If possible, duck into the lounge and try to speak to some waiting parents. Ask what they like about the place and what they think could be improved. You'll get straight info. Just be mindful that it may not be a good time for that parent. Trust your instincts.

CHAPTER 6 POP QUIZ ANSWERS

1. If you live in the U.S., the odds that your child will be hospitalized this year are . . . The answer is B, an unnerving 1 in 25. (Page 201.)

2. Before you check your child (or anyone else) into a hospital, you should make sure it's accredited by . . . The answer is D, The Joint Commission. (Page 200.)

3. Which statement best describes teaching hospitals? The answer is B; they are top-notch facilities that also train new doctors. (Page 205.)

4. Which of the following is the name of an anti-abduction system used in many hospitals? The answer is A, HUGS, an electronic monitoring bracelet system. (Of course, there are other good electronic anti-abduction systems out there; HUGS is just one that I know personally.) (Page 210.)

5. What is a common visual tool that good hospitals use to help children communicate their pain level? The answer is C, the Wong-Baker FACES scale. (Page 210.)

6. Which question should you ask before selecting a hospital to perform surgery on your child? The answer is D, all of the above. (Page 211.)

7. Which practice has been found to reduce the number of medication errors in hospitals by two-thirds? The answer is A, having a pharmacist on rounds. (Page 209.)

Chapter 7

At the Hospital...
Who's in Charge Here?

Making Sure the Lucky Staff
Will Never, Ever Forget You

POP QUIZ

How much do you know about navigating your way through a hospital stay and making sure your child has the safest hospital trip possible? Take the pop quiz below and find out. (Tip: There may be more than one correct answer.) If you get a perfect score, feel free to race on to the next chapter. Answers can be found at the end of the chapter.

1. When you learn that your child must be admitted to the hospital for any reason whatsoever, what's the first thing you should find out?
   A. How much this debacle is going to cost you
   B. Which items you're required to bring with you when your child checks in
   C. If your child can be an outpatient
   D. If your child can check in on a Monday, to avoid waiting for tests or other procedures all weekend

2. How many children in hospitals are injured by medical mistakes and adverse drug reactions every year?
   A. 1 in 15
   B. 1 in 5
   C. 1 in 2,200
   D. 1 in 90

3. Which of these phrases describes an ideal hospital stay?
    A. Convenient and special
    B. No muss, no fuss, no refunds
    C. Safe and memorable
    D. Quick and dull

4. Which of the following has been a key change in pediatric hospitals in the last three decades?
    A. Pediatric hospitals now require all parents to have some kind of medical training.
    B. Pediatric hospitals now refer to miniature straitjackets as "gentle restraints."
    C. Pediatric hospitals now encourage parents to sleep in the hospital so they can stay with their child.
    D. Pediatric hospitals now allow parents to stay with their child during surgery and even help administer the initial anesthesia to their child—under an anesthesiologist's careful supervision, of course.

5. According to regulations, how long must all hospital staffers wash their hands (with soap and water or an alcohol-based sanitizer) before and after contact with a patient?
    A. Ten seconds
    B. Fifteen seconds
    C. Thirty seconds
    D. Forty-five seconds

6. What should be your number one motto when your child is in the hospital?
    A. What Doesn't Kill You Only Makes You Stronger.
    B. Speak Up.
    C. Listen! You Don't Learn Much When You're Talking.
    D. To Make an Omelet, You Need to Break a Few Eggs.

In chapter 6, we laid out a plan to find the best hospital for your child when that need arises (odds are it will at some point). When you've completed that vital first step, you'll feel immensely reassured knowing that—if the time comes—your child will be in the best place possible. Next step: Knowing what to do after your kid is *in* the hospital and wearing that nifty wrist ID bracelet.

It's easy to be paranoid about hospitals. You've probably heard that an estimated ninety-eight thousand people die every year from medical errors, and that figure is likely far lower than the real total. Medical mistakes and adverse reactions to drugs injure one in fifteen hospitalized children, according to the journal *Pediatrics*. With all the media stories about errors, rampant infections, and "supergerms" crawling around, most parents might prefer to let their child drift across the English Channel in an inner tube rather than spend a week in the hospital. Any hospital stay offers a rich dose of irony: Your child has never been in better hands or faced more possible risks. Which way that scale tips depends on many factors. Some you can't control, but the majority you can *if* you take charge at the hospital—nicely, respectfully, appropriately, but definitely. It's the only way to ensure your child receives VIP (Very Important Patient) care.

Yes, I know, every patient should get that kind of care. But guess what? It doesn't always happen. No matter how brilliant, meticulous, and super-qualified the hospital team, *you* need to make sure that everything goes smoothly. Your child's chances for successful treatment increase greatly if you take control.

Your Best Defense:
An Insider's Game Plan

As a doctor and a mom, I have to let you in on an unnerving reality: You won't be able to protect your child from all the risks in a hospital. Even if you could zip your kid into a three-foot hazmat suit at check-in, it simply isn't possible to watch over every bit of care your child will receive. But if you're armed with my in-

Quick and Dull

That may not be the ideal motto for other aspects of your life, but it's the perfect description of a fantastic hospital stay, whether the patient is a newborn or the Pope. You want to get in and out as quickly as possible without a single memorable moment to tell your friends. Boring. That's your goal.

sider's game plan, you can maximize your child's chances of a safe, successful visit while minimizing the odds that you'll go insane.

Warning: This game plan requires gumption, nerve, chutzpah, and sometimes repeating yourself to an annoying degree. Know that up front. When your kid's in the hospital, there is no time to be meek. You'll need to be a cool-headed extrovert who can ask questions, complain when necessary, and still keep it together under pressure. (That includes being polite to all hospital staff.) You need to put your anxieties aside and bring your take-charge attitude front and center.

The Perks of Same-Day Service

Your first mission? **Ask if your child can be an outpatient.** Happily, pediatric medicine has evolved to the point where same-day surgery is now common for many procedures that used to require a night or five in the hospital. These include tonsillectomies, ear-tube surgery (myringotomy), and hernia repairs. In addition to better surgical techniques, we can thank newer, short-acting anesthesia that allows patients to walk out of the hospital hours after surgery. If your child can be treated and released in the same day and sleep in his own (freshly laundered) bed that night, *everyone will be happier*.

I would opt for outpatient treatment for my own children whenever it's possible and medically wise. It's not that I mind sacking out in a makeshift bed in a hospital ward (as an intern and resident, I certainly got used to doing that on marathon shifts). My beef comes down to math: Every hour any child spends in a hospital increases the risk that *something will go wrong*. Your child could pick up a nasty infection from a rogue supergerm or get the wrong treatment or drug. While it's good to know that the vast majority of errors don't result in serious problems, they can slow healing or cause extra pain or discomfort for your child—and extra stress for you, too. Getting in and out as quickly as possible is the best strategy.

Less stress, fewer risks, lower costs . . . getting top-notch hospital care on an outpatient basis is almost always a win-win-win.

That said, if your child *needs* to stay in the hospital overnight or longer, don't freak. It can be the best place for kids who require hospital-strength care and attention.

Getting Through Admissions

Whether your child will be in the hospital for three hours or three weeks, you'll need to go through some form of admission process. So let's talk about it.

For outpatient situations, most hospitals now pre-register you over the phone a day or two before. This lets you handle a lot of the paperwork and insurance issues in advance. Some hospitals now have videos you can watch at home so that you get up to speed on the exact procedure being done. This will cut down on your anxiety because you'll know what to expect. The day of the procedure, you will check in your child, who'll get a plastic ID bracelet with his name, date of birth, food or drug allergies, and medical record number.

Outpatient procedures tend to move swiftly. Once your child is settled in, your physician will go over what's being done and the risks involved. You will be asked to sign an "informed consent" form, which states that you understand the risks and benefits of the treatment your child is having. As you probably suspect, these forms can be hard to read and even tougher to understand. (I've often wondered which would be more useful in deciphering them: a law degree or fluency in hieroglyphics.) Luckily, things are beginning to improve in this respect—see "When Forms Attack," below.

When Forms Attack

 If you've ever had a close brush with medical paperwork, this won't surprise you a bit:

* Most patients **don't** read the forms they're given before having surgery or medical treatment. They just sign them.
* More than half of those who DO read the forms don't understand them.
* Only **one-fourth** of forms include all the data necessary to make an informed decision.

Most people just give this mountain of legalese a cursory scan, glaze over, and sign where directed—hoping that the hospital hasn't buried anything too outrageous in the microprint.

But here's the thing: After my years in medicine, I would pore over those forms with a magnifying glass. And so should you. You not only need to understand what you're signing but you have a right to expect those forms to be understandable. And in a growing number of hospitals, they are. The Centers for Medicare and Medicaid Services are prodding hospitals to design patient-friendly informed-consent processes. Hospitals that don't comply could lose their eligibility to bill Medicare for treatments. The Joint Commission recommends both easy-to-read forms and "teach-back" methods in which the patient is asked to repeat back what he's been told about the risks and benefits. Even the Department of Veterans Affairs has a new system that's written at a sixth-grade level and covers more than two thousand procedures in thirty specialties.

Ideally, the hospital you choose will have easy-to-understand forms. **But don't sign anything you don't understand, and do ask for more information if something is unclear.** You don't want to find out unexpectedly that you just underwent a procedure that had a 10 percent long-term success rate—or get home and find that the hospital now holds the mortgage on your house.

What to Bring

The hospital's admissions person will tell you what to bring for your child's hospital stay—but just in case, here's my must-bring list:

- An up-to-date list of any medications, vitamins, supplements, and herbal and home remedies your child takes (bring the actual medications if that's easier). Give a copy to the pediatric nurse in charge, who must know *everything* your child takes.

- A pair of slippers or flip-flops to keep germs off your kid's feet—and bed. You may also want to bring your child's own pajamas or robe. Some kids are happy (even giddy) to wear a hospital gown—doctor-sanctioned mooning comes but rarely in life—but other children may find that wearing their own PJs makes them feel better.
- Toiletries
- Clothes to go home in (a loose T-shirt or button-up-the-front top, if that makes it easier to get dressed after surgery)
- A favorite teddy bear or blanket, favorite drinking cup or bottle, or other comfort items—really, anything that will make the visit feel more like home
- Toys, videos, books, and games—most hospitals will have these, but I'd also bring my own from home. You don't know who's been touching a hospital's toys or how often they're cleaned.

There are also three things you should pack for yourself:

- A notebook. Use it to write down the names and titles of your health care team and details about tests, medications, and procedures. This will let you keep everything in one place. It's also a good way to start a detailed medical record for your child if you don't have one yet.
- Your cell phone—charged up, of course
- Your own favorite pillow or throw or anything that will help you sleep at night

What About Your Accommodations?

Most parents want to spend the night in the hospital with their young child. This is often best for everyone (see "How Will This Affect My Child?" on page 230). But make sure you get an early start on this; overnight spots for parents are often limited and fill up quickly. Well ahead of check-in, ask what accommodations the hospital has, whether one or both parents may stay, and what to bring along.

Comfort varies. In certain hospitals, "overnight accommodations" might be a vinyl armchair. In others, you'll have a relatively comfortable place to bed down. But even if your back doesn't love sleeping on a rollaway bed, pullout couch, or reclining chair, remember that your child will feel safer and more secure with you right there. And you can remind him of your selflessness decades from now when he fusses about taking two hours out of his day to drive you to the doctor.

Preparing Your Child

If it's not an emergency—and if it is, flip back to chapter 5—you should have time to prepare your child before going to the hospital. When and what should you say? Or not say? The answers depend on your child's age and the medical situation.

You can find good age-appropriate books on prepping your child at a library or bookstore. Below are three I recommend for younger kids; you'll find plenty more (for helping your child deal with everything from a hospital stay to learning to swim) in *Books to Grow With: A Guide to Using the Best Children's Fiction for Everyday Issues and Tough Challenges* by Cheryl Coon (Lutra Press, 2004):

- *Miffy in the Hospital* by Dick Bruna (Kodansha America, 2000, for ages three to eight)
- *Paddington Bear Goes to the Hospital* by Michael Bond and Karen Jankel (HarperCollins Juvenile Books, 2001, for ages four to eight)
- *Franklin Goes to the Hospital* by Paulette Bourgeois (Scholastic, 2000, for ages four to eight; also available in Spanish).

Infants

While getting any medical care for an infant is scary, you're actually getting off pretty easy as far as planning goes. Why? Two biggies: First, your ten-week-old isn't accustomed to long talks yet and will be ready to go to the hospital the minute you are. Second, you can spend most of your energy making sure that the hospital is ready for your infant—and that you and your family are prepared to handle the schedule complications even a short hospital stay will bring.

On the downside, expect your baby to be upset when you get to a big, busy, clinical place and she senses this isn't her auntie's house. So your already stressful day may be accompanied by that classic soundtrack "Endlessly Screaming Baby." Remind yourself that it's *normal* for infants to cry. I know that it's not easy to hear (for parents and innocent bystanders alike), but crying is how your little one communicates discomfort or fear. And she'll have plenty of both, since you're taking her to a strange environment with strange people, startling sounds, and harsh smells. Honestly, if the odor of hospital disinfectant nearly makes *you* want to cry, just imagine how she feels.

Try not to wear fear on your face; infants pick up on that. You might not believe it, but staying calm can be the biggest help to your baby. Ask hospital staffers about specific concerns or worries you have if it helps you stay steady.

Toddler/Preschooler (Ages One to Four)

One thing you have going for you at this age: Attention spans are quite short. Little kids live for the moment and don't dwell on the future—even if the future is, say, about three hours from now. However, not all toddlers are alike. Some four-year-olds are more intuitive and insightful than their twelve-year-old siblings.

So gear all of your explanations, descriptions, and assurances about the hospital stay to your child's individual development level. Some tips:

- The day before you leave for the hospital, take ten minutes (max) to tell your child where he is going, why, and what will happen, but be a little skimpy on the details. Tell the truth, but skip words like "scalpel," "knife," "needle," "slice," "saw," "cut off," or "fry." If he asks, "Will I get a shot?" a good reply would be, "I don't know, but if the doctor does have to give you one, I promise to make her do it fast so it hurts only a little."
- Do not tell your child that he won't feel a thing because the doctor will put him "to sleep." Many kids are afraid that they'll go the way of a sick dog or cat (complete with being buried under the bushes behind the garage). Instead, explain that the medicine will make him so sleepy that he won't feel or remember anything. You can tell your child you will be with him when he gets the medicine and that once the medicine wears off, he will wake up to find you right there at his bedside. (Naturally, you'd better be there. An ill-timed bathroom break could cost you big-time.)
- If your child asks how long the operation will take, put it in terms he will understand, like "about as long as your favorite TV show."
- Have your child help you pack the suitcase, and let him throw in things like toys and blankets for comfort. If he's going in for surgery, your child will usually be able to bring a "comfy" into the operating room to calm him before he's given anesthesia. Then the staff will discreetly stash it so it doesn't affect the sterile environment.
- Talk about the future. Tell him he'll feel better afterward and start planning a special treat together for when you get home.
- Be ready to repeat any of the above several times during the car trip and again in the hospital.

Kids Five to Nine Years Old

A lot of your prep work will be constantly saying that everything will be *okay*. From your child's view, he's going to a place filled with big equipment, creepy noises, a strange bed, and people he doesn't know—and, unlike a three-year-old, he's old enough to take these pretty seriously. No wonder he's scared. The key is to be honest and include your child in preparations. Some tips:

- If your child is five to seven, start talking about the hospital visit about three days beforehand, depending on his individual development. If your child is eight to ten, you may want to bring it up sooner, depending on his maturity level and attention span. Just don't talk about the hospital so much that you make your child anxious about it.
- Focus on the purpose of the trip: to help him get better and back home as soon as possible.
- Your child is smart, so be as straightforward as you can and give him permission to be a little upset or cry. If you're painting an overly rosy picture, he'll detect it—even if he doesn't call you on it.
- Use terms your child understands when describing what will happen in the hospital. As long as it won't scare your child or gross her out, consider using visuals, such as pictures from an anatomy book, to show your child the body part involved. The hospital may have a video of the procedure that is geared to kids.
- Stress the positive outcome expected from the procedure. Remind your child that he will feel better when it's over and soon be able to get back to his favorite activities. And let him know that he'll also have a treat waiting for him—at this age, maybe a new video game or a week without having to clean up his room.

Adolescent/Teen (Ten and Up)

Starting around age ten, kids will have a *lot* of questions and fears about any medical treatment. And they'll have misconceptions from a hodgepodge of sources. They may have seen plenty of gross things on the Discovery Health Channel. Or autopsy animations on *CSI*. Or been hooked on *Scrubs*. Given this, you'll be walking a fine line between being honest and open and sharing too much information. At the same time, it's difficult to hide scary stuff from preteens and teens; they can jump on the Internet at school or at home and find a colossal amount of info about anything—not all of it helpful or correct.

What's going on inside your child's head? Preteens and teens fear *pain, disfigurement,* and *losing control* (all worthy of fear, I'd say). The fear of being labeled a "freak" by their peers can be the fourth big dramatic deal and shoot to the top of the list at any given moment. Being in a hospital for any reason can signal to kids that they are "sick" and different at a time when they desperately want to fit in. Here are some ways to help adolescents and teens prepare:

- Explain the procedure and the reason for it. Use videos if possible—many hospitals now offer online links you can watch that demonstrate the procedure. Talk about the benefits and about feeling better when it's over. Tell the truth but remember that you're talking to a nervous child—don't go overboard and speak to him as if he's grown-up. Even if he's a mature fifteen and acts like an adult in many ways, right now he's looking to you for reassurance.
- Don't "open up" about your own fears or anxieties. Your child needs to rely on you right now and not see you as a nervous wreck or worry about *your* well-being.
- Adolescents tend to worry about waking up in the middle of the operation, so assure your child that this won't happen. If he searches on the Internet and finds out that the odds

of this happening are extremely low *but not nil,* have the anesthesiologist talk him through it.

- Encourage your child to ask doctors and nurses questions. This will make him feel empowered and also hopefully clear up any misconceptions about pain or disfigurement.
- If your kid's facing a slow recovery or dealing with a long-term problem, find a support group that will help your child meet others with similar experiences.

How Will This Affect My Child?

If a hospital stay when you were a kid was the most traumatic experience of your life, don't assume that your child will face the same ordeal—or be saddled with the same cold-sweat nightmares that you took home. Even as little as twenty years ago, we knew relatively little about how deeply a hospital stay could affect a child. Given this, kids were often left alone—their parents couldn't stay overnight, and visiting hours were rigidly limited. Parents thought they were doing the right thing by leaving, but—surprise—researchers now say that some kids were traumatized by the hospital experience and felt their parents had let them down. If you were hospitalized as a kid, maybe you can relate to this.

Fortunately, things have changed dramatically for the better. Most hospitals now allow at least one parent to stay with their child twenty-four hours a day, no sneaking required. The exception is during the actual surgery—be thankful for that—but you can return to your child's side in the recovery room. As she awakens, she will assume you never left. (It'll help if you're wearing the same clothes.)

After the hospital experience is over, you may find that your child is fussy or ill behaved, has nightmares, cries, throws tantrums, refuses to eat, becomes withdrawn, or even starts sucking his thumb or wetting the bed. This is normal; it's a reaction to the stress. Highly stressed parents have been known to exhibit similar behaviors.

Most kids who are loved and well cared for will get past these issues soon, but tell your pediatrician if these symptoms linger. Hospital social workers and child life specialists (see page 212 for more on this useful professional) can help, too.

Keeping Family Life Going

Having a kid in the hospital will test the entire family. Doctor visits, lab tests, and frequent checkups will throw off everyone's regular schedule. There will be missed family meals, skipped soccer games, extra carpooling, hurt feelings, and a plethora of stress. To offset some of these pressures, plan ahead and reach out to family and friends. Take them up on their offers to help (if they didn't offer, no holiday newsletter for them). Having people to run errands, help with driving, and watch your other children during the disruption can be amazingly helpful. If someone has a nice, hot meal waiting for you at home, even better.

Get over any guilt. If you're like most moms and dads I know, you're a giving person and would help out a neighbor or friend with a sick child in a moment, so be open to receiving help this time. Remember, it's impossible to do it all yourself. And you'll have plenty of chances to return these favors. Parental union by-laws demand it.

Don't forget to alert teachers and counselors at your children's schools; they can smooth out potential hassles due to missed time and, more important, act as your eyes and ears, watching for any behavior changes or signs of stress among your other children. Make sure, too, that you and your spouse take care of yourselves and try (*try;* that's all I'm saying) to get enough rest and eat properly.

Who's Who in the Hospital?

After your child checks in, you'll be introduced to several hospital staffers who will complement the efforts of your pediatrician, surgeon, and/or specialist. You'll wonder what they do and why most of them are wearing clogs. (They hose off easily.) Below are some of the players you're likely to encounter:

Physicans

- **Interns:** Say hello to the newest of the new doctors—young physicians right out of medical school and in their first year of training. Under supervision, they can assist in operations and provide hands-on care to patients. Interns are also called first-year residents.
- **Residents:** These doctors have completed their internships, but they are still in training for their specialty (dermatology, pediatrics, etc.). Residencies can run from two to seven years, depending on the specialty, and residents are ranked by seniority: Junior residents are the newest; senior residents get to boss the junior residents around.
- **Fellows:** They act as the attending physician's right-hand doc. Fellows have already completed an internship and residency in a specialty—such as pediatrics—but are doing more training to specialize even further, such as becoming a pediatric cardiologist. Fellows report a patient's progress and issues to the attending physician and are usually available to the staff 24/7. Fellows are great sources of information about what's going on with your child.
- **Attending physicians:** Your child's attending physician is the one in charge—the doctor who makes the decisions about your child's care, even though other staff docs will participate in it. "The attending" is the decider. The attending may be your pediatrician if he or she has privileges at that hospital.

Nurses

- **Nurse's aides or nursing assistants:** Nurse's aides usually tend to bedside needs of patients and assist with routine tasks such as observing and recording vital signs. They also empty bedpans, bathe patients, stock supplies, and help with other essential tasks, such as keeping rooms clean. A nurse's aide or nursing assistant generally receives a degree as either a certified nurse assistant (CNA) or state-tested nurse aide (STNA).
- **Nurses:** They're the people who will care for your child most frequently. They administer medications, take vital readings, and do a thousand other things to make sure all treatment orders are being followed, nothing is going wrong, and your child is as comfortable as possible. Nurses are usually the most accessible caregivers; turn to them first with requests, questions, or problems.
- **Nurse managers:** As the title implies, these nurses manage the other nurses on a floor or in a department. If you're not happy with something and have repeatedly asked a nurse or nurse's aide to remedy the problem, ask to see the nurse manager.

Other Health Care Professionals You May Encounter

- **Nurse practitioners:** A nurse practitioner has a master's degree in nursing and received special training in performing physical exams, taking medical histories, and making basic diagnoses. If nurse practitioners encounter a complicated medical problem, they're trained to consult with the doctor.
- **Physician assistants:** Growing in numbers, physician assistants are licensed to practice medicine under the direct—or in some cases indirect—supervision of a physician. Most physician assistants receive a master's degree in either physician assistant studies (MPAS), health science (MHS), or medical science

(MMSc), which requires two to three years of training after receiving a bachelor's degree.

- **Physical therapists:** Generally, physical therapists (PTs) work during and/or after hospital stays to improve an injury or a condition such as cerebral palsy. They often achieve amazing results by exercising, stretching, and/or massaging the body. PTs focus on building strength, mobility, and flexibility as well as large motor skills.
- **Technicians:** Hospital tests are often run by technicians who specialize in doing certain kinds of procedures, such as taking

Little Things Mean a Lot

Remember that little things—besides keeping favorite toys within reach—can be big deals. These easy insider moves can make a hospital adventure more pleasant (okay, less rotten) for your child.

* **Ask the nurse to always apply numbing gel** before your child gets a shot or has blood drawn. Do you know that flavored medicine that dentists apply to your gums before giving a Novocain injection, so the needle won't hurt? A similar med can save your tyke a hundred ouches. Ask the nurse to apply EMLA or lidocaine cream to your child's skin about an hour before a scheduled needle stick.
* **Set limits.** Tell the nurses or interns that if they are unable to draw blood or insert an IV after two attempts, you would like another person to try.
* **If your child has to wear a surgical mask, have it lined with flavored Chapstick.** Cherry, of course.

ultrasounds or X-rays. They are responsible for doing the test correctly, not for interpreting the results, so don't ask them for those. A doctor will explain the results to you.

Six Tips to Grease the Wheels

Now that you know the key staff members, put this knowledge to use. Think of them as new friends who can play a critical role in your child's well-being—and can magically smooth out bumps and delays that plague less savvy parents and patients. Use these tips to reap strategic benefits:

1. **Ask staffers what they do.** It's hard to tell who's who based on their outfits—that impressive gentleman in the tie might be here to fix a broken dialysis machine. If you're not sure, just ask. Is the person a resident, intern, doctor, nurse, or nurse's aide? Any staffers who enter your child's room should have an ID badge on and say why they're there. (Refrain from yelling, "Halt! State your business!") By the way, they should also check your child's ID bracelet to make sure they have the right patient.

2. **Be extra nice to the nurses.** They are the workhorses, and they can make life for you and your child a whole lot easier, whether you need a washcloth, more pain medication, or face time with the doctor. Nurses get the brunt of abuse from angry patients and frustrated family members. Try saying "please," "thank you," and "I appreciate your help." You might be amazed by the attention you get.

3. **Be there when the nurses change shifts.** Nurses generally work twelve-hour shifts, and shift changes are often when mistakes get made in the hospital. Learn who the next nurse on duty is, and personally relay any important information about your child. Yes, the new nurse should

Speak Up!

You can't be a silent bystander at any point in the care of your child. Make sure to speak up if you have questions or concerns. If you're the shy, passive type, you need to go through a major personality change while your child is hospitalized. You are your child's advocate, and you need to take charge and communicate effectively with the hospital staff. You can't be afraid to ask questions or point out things that seem amiss.

To encourage patients and their families to do this, The Joint Commission has a campaign based upon two words. You guessed it: "speak up." This patient safety campaign is aimed at giving patients and their caregivers the muscle to prevent medical errors and infection. The Speak Up™ campaign has many suggestions for ways you can help prevent errors in your child's care. Here are a few:

* Don't be afraid to tell the staff if you think your child is about to get the wrong test or medication.
* If a worker isn't wearing gloves and is about to take your child's blood or other sample, say something. Also, the worker should always check your child's ID and ask for her birthday or other identifying information before any test or procedure. (Make sure the sample is labeled in front of you with your child's name on it.)

Many more Speak Up tips are available at www.jointcommission.org/PatientSafety/SpeakUp/

read the previous nurse's notes, but don't rely only on that. Remember that the nurse may have more patients to care for than just your child.

4. **Know the shortcuts.** Get friendly with the resident or intern so you can get quick answers to relatively basic questions. Both should have access to the attending physician and will likely get back to you with an answer faster than you'd be able to track the attending physician down. Of course, for important questions, ask to see the attending personally.

5. **If an intern explains test results and you have questions,** it's fine to ask a resident, fellow, or attending physician how they interpret the results. Some findings are very clear, such as "Your test results are normal." But others may require lengthier discussions, so it's always okay to ask.

6. **Start every day nudging.** Every morning, your first question for the attending physician or resident should be, "What's the *specific plan* for today?" This can subtly prod them to keep things moving. You don't want to wait five days for tests that could be completed in two.

Wash Your Hands! Please!

This isn't just a request. **It's a commandment.** It should be chiseled on a massive granite block in every pediatric department—make that *every* department—in every hospital in the world. (Yes, that's a lot of granite, but that's how important this is.)

All hospital staffers must WASH THEIR HANDS before treating your child and before touching any object that may come in contact with your child.

Guess who must enforce this commandment? That's right. You. *Make sure* that everyone washes with soap and warm water or uses a hand sanitizer before they touch your child. *(This goes for you, too.)* Hand washing is the single most effective way to keep your child from picking up an infection that could be life threatening. It's not an idle precaution: Hospitals that successfully increase hand washing see their infection rates drop.

If it's so basic and sensible, why do you have to worry about making sure doctors and nurses wash their hands?

Because hospital staffers forget to do it. Constantly.

Studies estimate that hand-washing rates in hospitals average 40 percent to 60 percent on *"a good day."* One study found that medical students washed their hands most often, while surgeons, anesthesiologists, and critical-care doctors washed their hands least often. Not what you want to hear, right? That's why you have to be the cop. You might have to repeat "Please wash your hands" so often while your child is in the hospital that you start mumbling it in your sleep.

Now, I know it's not always easy to say, "Excuse me, doctor, but please wash your hands or use the sanitizing gel before touching my child." It can feel like you're criticizing or being bossy. But it's every staffer's obligation to do so and *your right to demand it.* Some parents are squeamish about mentioning hand hygiene to harried doctors and nurses for fear of aggravating them. Don't be. Because here's the harsh reality: If you wimp out on insisting that all staffers wash their hands, you're endangering your child's life.

First of all, your child is already vulnerable to the garden-variety bacteria and viruses that all humans spread during physical contact—and even ordinary bugs can be deadly when a child is already weakened by illness. Second, hospitals are *filled* with powerful germs that can cause severe, difficult-to-treat infections. Probably the most famous is MRSA (methicillin-resistant *Staphylococcus aureus*), which is a much hardier variation of the common "staph" bacterium (see page 11 for more details). Unlike typical staph—which can also be deadly to very ill patients—MRSA has developed a resistance to so many antibiotics that doctors have a hard time killing it. That's why it's often called a superbug. MRSA is rampant in hospitals, nursing homes, and other health care centers where people have weakened immune

The Fifteen-Second Rule

Did you know that there's a national regulation stipulating how long hospital staffers must wash their hands? Workers are required to use alcohol-based hand sanitizers or soap and warm water for at least ~~fifteen seconds~~ before and after every direct contact they have with a patient, with bodily excretions, or with contaminated surfaces or objects. Fifteen seconds, just so you know, is about the time it takes to sing all four lines of the "Happy Birthday" song. Feel free to use this as a trivia question.

systems. Frighteningly, MRSA infection rates in hospitals are rising throughout the world.

The fortunate (and sad) thing? It's fairly easy to prevent MRSA, and other bugs too, from attacking your child. The first step is the obvious one: religious hand washing. Second, and just as important, is making certain that *medical equipment isn't contaminated.* Any piece of equipment that touches your child (such as a stethoscope) should be wiped with alcohol before use, unless the staffer just took it out of a sterile container. **One big tip:** If your child needs an IV, make sure it is inserted and removed under clean conditions—ideally, in a designated treatment room by a gloved nurse. The skin should be cleaned with alcohol and/or Betadine solution before the IV is inserted, and the IV should be changed at least every three to four days.

Where's Your Sign?

External prompts—signs—can be a big help in (tactfully) reminding hospital workers about hand hygiene. For example, The Joint Commission distributes pins for hospital staffers to wear that read, "Ask me if I washed my hands." I also see many wise patients post large, marker-drawn signs on their room door and near their bed that read, "Have you washed your hands?" and "Have you washed your stethoscope?" Many people also bring in a huge jug of alcohol-based sanitizing gel from a drugstore or warehouse wholesale store and place it next to the hospital bed, with a label reading, "Please Use Me!" These are easy ways of reminding doctors, nurses, and other hospital personnel about their obligation, and it will break the ice during those moments when you may feel a little awkward about ordering a brusque offender to scrub up. One glance at your signage will let all peo-

Have a Complaint?

If you have a complaint about the care your child received while at the hospital, you should file a complaint with the organization itself. Additionally, if the hospital is accredited by The Joint Commission, contact The Joint Commission's Office of Quality Monitoring via e-mail at complaint@jointcommission.org or by fax at (630) 792-5636. You can also call (800) 994-6610 if you have a question about how to file your complaint. You can provide your contact information or submit a complaint anonymously if you prefer. Find more information here: www.jointcommission.org/GeneralPublic/Complaint/oqm.htm.

ple know you're highly sensitive—and perhaps appropriately neurotic—about hand washing, so they will have no right to bristle if they ignore the signs and force you to *verbally* ask them to wash.

The bottom line and last word on this critical issue: If anyone rolls their eyes or balks at your constant insisting that all staffers wash their hands—which should never happen but unfortunately might—don't back down. They'll respect you for it. You can bet that if they were the one in the hospital bed, they'd be twice as insistent!

Three Common Surgeries

Scene: two parents waiting in the pediatric surgery lounge. One says, "What brings you here?" I'd be willing to bet my favorite pair of shoes that the other parent replies with one of three answers:

Hernia. Tonsillectomy. Or ear tubes.

If you can get through parenthood without having a child who needs to have a hernia repaired, tonsils/adenoids removed, or ear tubes surgically inserted, consider yourself lucky. Not $800 million Powerball lottery lucky, but lucky. These are *very* common procedures. Let's look at each.

1. Repairing Hernias

Babies can be born with hernias. And trust me, they're not lifting heavy furniture in the womb. A hernia occurs when a part of an organ or tissue pushes through a weak spot in the muscle wall and protrudes outward. The most serious kind is a strangulated hernia. This is when the blood supply is cut off from the protruding tissue, which becomes discolored or black and extremely painful. This is an emergency situation! Surgery is required *im-*

mediately to free the tissue so that oxygen-containing blood can get to it again.

Intermittent hernias—those that come and go—are much more common. If you see a little bulge of any kind in the groin area (called an inguinal hernia) or the belly-button area (called an umbilical hernia) that wasn't there the last time you looked, take a photo of it and bring the picture to the doctor's office since these intermittent hernias may not be visible during an exam. (You may also be able to e-mail a digital photo to your doctor's office.)

Umbilical hernias often don't require treatment. Most close by age one without any intervention, and nearly all close by age five. Still, doctors will often suggest surgery if the hernia gets bigger as your child grows or is present after age three. And inguinal hernias can be easily pushed back in with minor surgery—the procedure is often performed on an outpatient basis, though infants may be kept overnight. Most kids who have surgery feel better within a week.

2. Removing Tonsils and Adenoids

If your child has persistent tonsillitis, multiple strep infections, chronic sinusitis, sleep apnea, trouble breathing, or difficulty eating from swollen tonsils, your doctor may recommend removing the tonsils and/or adenoids. The surgery can be performed with a scalpel or with one of the newer laser techniques, which have cut total healing time down to a few days. Both require general anesthesia, meaning that your child will be "asleep" for about twenty to forty minutes. In-hospital recovery usually takes another five to ten hours, and then your child may be released. If he's under three or has a chronic disease, the surgeon may recommend an overnight stay. Depending on the technique used, your child will have a bad sore throat for several days and may also be tired from the anesthesia. Complete recovery usually takes about

Q: I had a tonsillectomy when I was seven. Shouldn't my child just get her tonsils removed, too?

A: Just because you spent four days in bed eating ice cream as a kid doesn't mean your child needs to experience this once-universal ritual. We do far fewer tonsillectomies today than docs did decades ago. Why? We're better at treating tonsillitis, for starters. Also, rather than just considering them a nuisance, we now know that tonsils help fight infection, so we make a big effort to leave them in their original home whenever possible.

But if your child constantly gets strep infections or tonsillitis, or wakes up gasping from sleep apnea (she may have nightmares in which she can't breathe—because she can't!), then, yes, she might need tonsil surgery. But not necessarily a full tonsillectomy. Today, we can surgically "shave" tonsils or use lasers to remove small amounts of tissue rather than always going for the full monty.

At least the ice cream part hasn't changed.

a week. Surgery on the adenoids is similar. Soft foods (read: ice cream and pudding) can soothe the pain from the surgery a bit.

3. Inserting Ear Tubes

Many, many kids between the ages of six months and two years get middle ear infections (otitis media). These infections are often treated with antibiotics, but if your child has repeated infections or starts to have hearing, speech, or developmental delays due to

Three Ways to Prevent Ear Infections
and Fluid in the Ears

1. Don't smoke around your child.
2. Don't bottle-feed children when they are in a
   horizontal position.
3. Avoid contact with others who are sick.

persistent fluid behind the eardrum, your pediatrician may recommend ear-tube surgery. I recently read that two million tubes are placed in children in the U.S. every year, and that figure doesn't shock me. It's an extremely common procedure. Placing small "tympanostomy tubes" in the eardrums helps equalize the pressure between the middle ear and the outer ear, which allows fluid or pus to drain out and relieves pressure and pain. While the tubes have to be inserted under general anesthesia, the whole process only takes about ten to fifteen minutes, and there's a good chance that your child will recover easily and leave the hospital in just a few hours.

Four Strategies to Make Surgery Easier

Surgery can scare the heck out of kids, just as it can scare adults. These four strategies can reduce fear and ease the journey for both you and your child.

1. Put on your game face. I've said this before but it bears repeating: For some parents, the hardest part of their child's surgery is trying not to fall apart themselves. But your child will be looking to you to see how you're doing, so you've got to be supportive, loving, sympathetic, and above all, *calm.* Even if you're a basket case, put on a happy face, hold hands with your child, and show him that you're confident that the outcome will be positive and everything will go as expected. If you need help getting yourself through this, contact the hospital's social worker and ask for tips.

2. Banish any misplaced guilt. Young children sometimes secretly believe that their medical problem and the operation is a form of punishment for being bad. Reassure your child that this problem is *not* the result of anything he or she did. Even if the problem might have been prevented—say, a bike accident when your son wasn't wearing his helmet—lay off the lectures until well *after* his surgery. Say, in a week or two. He doesn't need the extra stress of feeling guilty when he's having an operation and trying to recover.

3. Take a tour. Many hospitals have pre-op tours for children so they can try on a surgical mask, dress up in a hospital gown, handle a stethoscope, and see the kind of bed they will be in. Getting a glimpse of the hospital can take away the fear of the unknown. Your child will see that the staff is friendly and that there are other kids in the hospital who are coming and going.

4. Practice coping skills. The day you arrive, a child life specialist or social worker may teach your child calming skills, such as deep breathing and positive mental imagery, but you can practice those at home before you arrive, too. Provide lots of praise and support. During recovery, your child may feel pain or discomfort, and it helps to have ways to offset those feelings and even reduce the need for pain medications.

Know Your Anesthesia . . .

If your child asks, "Will they put me to sleep by hitting me on the head with a big hammer?" you need a better answer than, "Uh, no." Here are the forms of anesthesia your child may receive:

Local numbing is used for minor procedures, such as stitches or wart removal. It involves injecting a local anesthetic into the surgical area to block pain. The patient remains awake.

Regional anesthesia, such as an epidural, is used to numb a bigger area of the body, such as the legs. The anesthesiologist injects a numbing agent around major nerves to block pain. In kids, regional anesthesia may be given for procedures involving the abdomen, arms, or legs. The patient remains awake, but often children are also given a sedative to help them relax (see below).

Sedation, sometimes referred to as "twilight sleep," is used to relieve anxiety and/or pain during a procedure. If your child receives regional or even local anesthesia for a procedure, he will be awake for it, but a sedative will likely be combined with the anesthesia to improve his comfort level—and decrease his squirminess.

General anesthesia is the out-cold variety. If your child needs surgery, the anesthesiologist will most likely recommend going this route because young children simply can't stay still during most operations, even relatively minor ones. The anesthesiologist administers the anesthesia through an IV drip and/or an inhaled gas. General anesthesia affects the brain as well as the entire body, so your child will not feel pain or remember the surgery. Know, too, that your child will have a breathing tube and be hooked up to a ventilator to assist him in breathing while under general anesthesia.

... And Know Your Anesthesiologist

Regardless of the type of anesthesia used, you and your child should meet with the anesthesiologist. (Hopefully, your hospital has a *pediatric* anesthesiologist who will be caring for your child.) Schedule this appointment a day or so before surgery, or earlier during the same day if it's an outpatient procedure. The two of you should have a thorough chat about your child's medical history and any special concerns.

What are the risks and dangers of anesthesia? Given today's safety standards, the life-threatening risks are very, very low. Your child may experience some side effects, which are generally mild, such as being disoriented, agitated, or nauseous. Vomiting, drowsiness, dizziness, and a sore throat are also pretty common. Most side effects either wear off or are treatable.

I'd opt for local anesthesia whenever possible, as it's the most mild, but it's often not practical for even minor surgeries on children due to the fidget factor.

Doctor, May I Have Your Autograph?

Before your child is wheeled away for surgery, ask the surgeon to mark the spot being operated on—especially if the procedure involves a right/left distinction between arms, legs, fingers, or toes, or if it involves a part of the body like the spine, which has multiple levels. ("Wrong-site errors" occur more frequently during spinal surgeries, by the way, because it's quite easy to operate on the wrong vertebrae or disk.)

Normal protocol is for the surgeon to write his or her initials (or the word "yes") on the surgical site. Surgeons don't use an "X" to mark the spot, since that could be construed as meaning "don't operate here." And that could lead to a big, bad goof. (By the way, this surgical site marking is required by The Joint Commission—which is good news for you.)

The Ins and Outs of Pain Medication

Kids hate pain. Adults aren't crazy about it either. That's one reason pain control is such a big part of any surgery or invasive procedure. Another reason is that uncontrolled pain can slow or even derail recovery; people who are in agony simply don't heal well and can suffer additional medical problems. What's more, they tend to make *very* unhappy patients, whether they're three or ninety years old. So hospital staffers take great pains to keep patients pain-free—or at least as comfortable as medically possible. Use these additional tips to make sure your child doesn't suffer unnecessarily:

- Before surgery, a nurse will probably give your child a mild sedative to make him relaxed and sleepy. Ask the doctor if your child should also receive **additional pain medication before or during the surgery** so it's already working when he wakes up in the recovery room.
- If your child's pain is severe, **ask to speak to a pain specialist** (usually a specially trained anesthesiologist).
- **Ask about nondrug pain relief,** including relaxation techniques such as deep breathing. Your doctor may also recommend heat or cold compresses, massage, rest, changing positions in bed, or simply good distractions (such as TV, video games, music, puzzles, or drawing).
- If your child needs to take pain medication for a while, **be certain that it's carefully monitored.** Every time a nurse comes in with medication, check the drug name, dose, and schedule (to make sure it's the right amount of the right drug at the right time). Keep tabs on your child's medication schedule so you can hunt down the nurse if a round gets skipped—or keep an extra dose from being administered.
- **Ask the doctor if your child needs a prescription pain medication or if an over-the-counter product will do the job.**

Sometimes, the best post-surgery pain relief comes from simple medications like acetaminophen (Tylenol) and ibuprofen (Motrin or Advil).

- **Learn the side effects of your child's pain medication,** so you'll know what to expect and what's a trouble sign. Luckily, sleepiness is the most common side effect from pain meds. But constipation is common too, unfortunately.
- **Tell the staff about any signs that your child is in pain,** meaning any little, unusual things he may do that only you would recognize. This is especially important if you can't always be at his bedside.
- Most important, **speak up if you think your child is in pain!** Far too often, I see kids suffer needlessly because they're not getting effective pain medication. Don't be chicken. Don't accept responses like "Some pain is normal." Ask if the dose can be increased or if another drug might work better.

Pain Myth Busters

"If my child is sleeping and not complaining, she's comfortable, right?"
Not necessarily. Some kids sleep as a way of shutting out pain. If your child is old enough to talk, *ask* if she is in pain rather than trying to guess. Or ask a nurse to get the Wong-Baker FACES Pain Rating Scale (see chapter 6) if a copy of this well-known pain scale isn't already next to your child's bed. Then have your child pick out the face that matches her pain level. It's remarkably accurate.

"Taking drugs for pain is a sign of weakness."
I occasionally see macho parents who feel this way, but I've noticed that it's far easier to have this opinion when *you're not the one in pain.* Ahem. Anyway, it's simply not true. Pain doesn't make a child hardier. The fact is, not treating pain can make

things worse. Less pain means less stress on the body and the mind, so healing occurs faster. If your child hurts less, he will be able to get up and move around sooner after the surgery. You want that to happen because it reduces the risk of post-op complications, such as pneumonia, infections, fever, and blood clots. Be aware that everyone experiences pain differently, even after the same procedure.

"It's easy for children to become addicted to pain medication." Taking pain meds for several days won't make your seven-year-old a prescription-drug junkie. If your child needs to take

Intensive Care: Get Involved

If your child will be in an intensive care unit (ICU) following surgery or treatment, here's a tip: Be there for bedside rounds every day. That's when doctors, nurses, respiratory therapists, nutritionists, and other medical staff arrive at the same time to examine and talk to the patient. Ask what time rounds usually occur, and make sure you're not out grabbing a cup of coffee then. It's a great way to get accurate, detailed information from your child's health care team. A recent study found that when parents get involved in bedside rounds, it decreases their anxiety and increases trust between the parents and staff. It's also a good way for the medical team to get information they need from you directly, instead of through nurses—and direct communication is always a good thing.

pain meds or sedatives for a longer period, your doctor will decrease the dose slowly to prevent any withdrawal symptoms.

"Children are typically overmedicated for pain while being hospitalized."
I disagree. If anything, research—and my own experience—shows that children are undertreated for pain in the hospital. Yet there are excellent, mild medications that help kids a great deal, though many are underutilized. Bottom line: There is *no* reason for children to be in pain.

Homeward Bound

Before you leave the hospital, the doctor should explain what normal healing and recovery will look like. **Be sure to get discharge instructions;** they should detail everything you need to know to help your child recuperate successfully at home and specify the date of your follow-up visit with the surgeon or your pediatrician (if that's missing, make the appointment). Be sure that your discharge instructions contain **a list of danger signs to watch for in your child.** This list should include the following: a fever above 101 degrees; unusual or excessive bleeding, pain, redness, or discharge from the surgical site; unusual lethargy; an inability to keep fluids down; and a loss of appetite. Discharge instructions should also include **information about any prescribed medications** that you will be administering at home. Finally, **don't leave without the name and phone number of the person to call** if you suspect there's a problem or have any questions at all. That person may not be your surgeon or pediatrician, so don't simply assume that. Check it. And get it all in writing. You can't remember everything.

Home never looked so good, did it?

WHAT GOES WRONG IN HOSPITALS—AND WHY

If there's any good news with children being hospitalized, it's that more studies are revealing what goes wrong and how—and knowing that is the first step to knowing how to fix it. Here are some recent key findings.

- One study of thirty-eight American children's hospitals found that the most frequent complications in their young patients were from **infections due to medical care, respiratory failure following surgery, and infections in the bloodstream after surgery (sepsis)**. What's troubling is that the research found that most of the complications were preventable—often simply by better hand washing, sterilization, and other safety techniques that reduce hospital infections.

- **Medication mistakes in hospitals** have also been under the microscope. According to a 2008 study, drug errors affect 540,000 hospitalized kids in the U.S. every year— far more than experts had estimated. Why is your child especially vulnerable to medication screwups in the hospital? Depending on how long he's there, there's a good chance that several different people will be swinging by his room and giving him a lot of different medications. *That's why you need to double- and triple-check to be sure that every pill, injection, IV drip, and inhaler he receives is indeed the correct drug and that it's administered properly and on time.*

  The most common problems were with pain medications and antibiotics—kids received the wrong drug, received the wrong dose, or reacted badly to a drug. While fortunately most of the errors and reactions didn't cause serious trouble, the study found that 22 percent were preventable.

  You can help here, too: Remember that if your child is al-

ready taking *any* medications or supplements, or has food allergies, it's vital for that information to get into the hospital's
records *and* to the head nurse. For life-threatening allergies,
be sure that your child wears a MedicAlert bracelet.

Six Ways to Keep a Medical Mistake from Happening to Your Child

These are excerpted from a patient tip sheet published by the
U.S. government. While all the info in it is useful, using this
little hospital checklist from Uncle Sam can go a long way to
keeping your kid out of medical trouble. (You can find the entire list, called "20 Tips to Help Prevent Medical Errors in Children," at www.ahrq.gov/consumer/20tipkid.htm.)

1. **If you have a choice, pick a hospital at which many chil-
    dren have the procedure your child needs.** As previously
    mentioned, *all* patients, young and old, tend to do better in
    hospitals that have a great deal of experience treating their
    condition. Ask how many of the procedures have been per-
    formed at the hospital.

2. **Make sure you know who is in charge of your child's care
    at the hospital.** This will be the attending physician—most
    likely a surgeon or specialist, not your pediatrician. Iden-
    tifying this person is especially important if your child has
    many health problems.

3. **Make sure that all health professionals involved in your
    child's care have important medical information about
    him.** Do not assume that everyone knows everything they
    need to.

4. **If you don't trust yourself to speak up, bring along some-
    one you do trust.** Ask a vocal family member or friend to

help be your child's advocate. This person can also help you remember instructions during what can be an over-whelmingly stressful period. Time to call in a few favors!

5. **Ask why each test or procedure is being done.** It is a good idea to find out why a test or treatment is needed and how it can help. Sometimes a test is optional and your child could be better off without it.

6. **When your child is being discharged from the hospital, go over the home treatment plan** *twice.* Research shows that at discharge time, doctors think people understand more than they really do about what they should and should not do when they return home.

Source: Agency for Healthcare Research and Quality, U.S. Department of Health and Human Services.

CHAPTER 7 POP QUIZ ANSWERS

1. When you learn that your child must be admitted to the hospital for any reason whatsoever, what's the first thing you should find out? The answer is C—whether you can go the outpatient route. It can make this adventure much easier on everyone and on your wallet, as well. (Page 220.)

2. How many children in hospitals are injured by medical mistakes and adverse drug reactions every year? The answer is A, 1 in 15. (Page 219.)

3. Which of these phrases describes an ideal hospital stay? The answer is D. If I had my druthers, I wouldn't want an iota of excitement or a single "memorable" moment during my child's hospital stay, believe me. (Page 220.)

4. Which of the following has been a key change in pediatric hospitals in the last three decades? The answer is C. Pull out that trundle bed . . . or do your darnedest to recline on that recliner. (Page 230.)

5. According to regulations, how long must all hospital staffers wash their hands (with soap and water or an alcohol-based sanitizer) before and after contact with a patient? The answer is B, at least fifteen seconds. That's about as long as it takes to sing the "Happy Birthday" song, by the way. (Page 239.)

6. What should be your number one motto when your child is in the hospital? The answer is B. Always, but always, *speak up*! (Page 236.)

Chapter 8

The Twenty Stickiest Questions I Get Asked

And Why You Should Avoid "Headline Parenting"

POP QUIZ

Like most docs, I answer many of the same questions over and over. Not that I mind—I love the teaching part of my job, and I love inquiring parents and curious kids (unless the *only* thing they say is "Why?"). But sometimes simple questions are anything but. Take this quiz to see if you can spot some of the stickiest questions and trickiest answers. If you miss a few, keep reading—good bet there is more you don't know. (And as always, there may be more than one correct response.) Answers can be found at the end of the chapter.

1. Which statement best describes the evidence about vaccines causing autism?
   - A. There's no clear cause-and-effect evidence.
   - B. It's shaky at best.
   - C. It's disturbing.
   - D. It's circumstantial but growing.

2. Do babies really need to sleep on their backs all the time?
   - A. Only if they are comfortable in that position
   - B. No, that's an old myth
   - C. Yes, to reduce the risk of SIDS
   - D. Only when they are running a fever

3. When using an insect repellent that contains DEET on a child, which strategy should you follow?
   A. Choose a repellent that has twice the DEET concentration that you think your child will need, to be safe.
   B. Apply it only once per day; when the protection time expires, head indoors.
   C. Reapply the repellent every few hours to make sure the protection remains strong.
   D. Use a product that combines sunscreen and insect repellent, to get dual coverage with fewer applications.

4. Transmission of Lyme disease from a tick may occur . . .
   A. If the tick has been attached to the body for twenty-four hours or more
   B. If when you try to remove the tick, the body comes off but the head remains attached
   C. If the tick is picked up within a hundred miles of Lyme, New Hampshire
   D. If the tick becomes extremely angry and agitated while sucking out blood

5. When should a child's blood levels of lead be tested?
   A. At eight to twelve months of age, and then every year through kindergarten
   B. Only after being exposed to a likely lead source, such as old, chipped paint
   C. Every three months if you live in an urban environment; every six months in a rural environment
   D. Children really don't need lead testing today; it's a vestige from the 1950s.

6. If you suspect that your child's persistent sore throat is caused by a strep infection, do you need to go to the pediatrician for a strep culture test?
   A. Yes
   B. No; just phone your pediatrician and request an antibiotic prescription.
   C. It's optional; if your pediatrician decides to prescribe antibiotics without ordering a culture test, that's fine.
   D. Maybe; try medicated lozenges first to see if the strep goes away on its own.

7. What does Dr. Jen personally think of sippy cups?
   A. They're wonderful. Every child should carry one, whenever possible.
   B. They're overused and likely contributing to obesity and tooth decay.
   C. They should only be used during car trips.
   D. They're perfectly fine as long as they're made in the U.S.A.

If you're a parent of a young child and lucky enough to get a chance to sit down in a rare moment—say, when no one's screaming or about to give what looks like a piece of the coffeemaker to the dog—don't spend the time flipping through a newspaper or watching the news. If you do, odds are that you'll find a short article in a newspaper about, say, an everyday food additive that has been associated with anemia in baby mice and should be removed from your kitchen *this very moment*. Or perhaps the network news anchor will inform you that your pediatrician just prescribed a potentially useless medication for your two-year-old—at least according to a small Norwegian study.

Like most good parents, you'll hop on the Internet to get more info.

Fifteen minutes later, you'll be calling Poison Control (1-800-222-1222), your pediatrician, 911, or the school nurse. Why? A well-intentioned online search about a pediatric health issue can quickly send anyone into a tizzy. You'll find dozens of websites—both credible and crazy—offering a smorgasbord of warnings. Did your doctor really give your baby *three vaccines* in one visit? Did you really schedule your child for a tonsillectomy? What were you thinking?

It would be easier if the people quoted on these websites were all obvious wackos. But some are respected physicians. Some are researchers at well-known universities. And many may be telling you to do exactly the opposite of what your pediatrician advises. What should you do?

Headline Parenting

Pediatrics (like medicine in general) is rife with controversy and conflicting opinions, usually over inconclusive information. Add in some bad mistakes in our medical history—such as thalidomide, a drug prescribed in the late 1950s and early 1960s to combat morning sickness in pregnant women that turned out to cause horrible birth defects in their children—and it's easy to see why skepticism and fear can unnerve even sensible, smart parents.

In many cases, you and other parents face a frustrating quandary: How can you be sure you're doing the right thing for your child when your pediatrician, specialists, hospital physicians, and health insurance company may not agree on what's best or even safe?

When parents try to navigate the floodwaters of health information (and misinformation) out there, they often end up overreacting to the latest scary news story. This causes a phenomenon called "headline parenting," which pediatricians, myself included, see in excess. After a scare story runs in the news, moms and dads will suddenly stop using baby formula, or cancel a vaccination, or banish all plastic food containers, or hurriedly enact some other plan that's a nuisance at best and dangerous at worst. When I'm lucky, parents will call me first, and I can help them sort out the sane advice from the needlessly scary or downright silly. For instance, quite often parents arrive with printouts of Web pages or magazine articles, which usually have frightening headlines, such as "Mercury in Tap Water," "DEET Causes Cancer," "Vaccines and Learning Disorders," and on and on. The titles are sometimes enough to scare *me*, even when I know an article or study has been discredited.

In some cases, a five-minute discussion will relieve a parent's fears. Other times, it's not so simple.

Grappling with Unknowns

Although I don't like saying it, sometimes "I don't know" is the only answer a doctor can give. My delivery, however, is more scientific than a shrug of the shoulders followed by "I dunno." You've probably heard a version of this: "We can't say for certain yet if the side effects from this medication, which occurred in 65 percent of the small study group, apply to larger populations, so more data is needed." In these "I don't know" situations, we always say, "More data is needed," because more data *is* needed.

The problem, of course, is that to parents this answer typically means "Do this, because right now it's the most logical thing to do, given the limited knowledge we doctors are working with. But we reserve the right to say 'Oops, sorry. We were wrong' tomorrow."

That's not very comforting. And that's why smart parents ask tough questions. Even when there are no "right" answers, partial answers are better than none. Getting the best possible information—and making a plan based on it, then changing course if it becomes necessary—is the goal that smart parents and pediatricians work together to achieve.

Sticky Questions

I field tough questions—the kind that may have no perfect answers—every day. Unless you handle them carefully and methodically, you can get tangled in an unholy mess of half science, conjecture, and what-ifs. They're sticky because while many do have fairly clear, straightforward answers, parents have a difficult time accepting them if 1) they're not the answers they want to hear, or 2) they've been misled by convincing but untrustworthy information or thinly disguised marketing hype.

Finally, they're sticky questions because they can turn a fifteen-minute office visit into a thirty-five-minute debate unless handled with care. I won't lie; there are times when I groan at the prospect of hashing through some of these issues, especially when it's clear that a parent already has a polarized opinion based on a two-minute TV news "report." But I quickly swallow my groan, since the opportunity to share what I know—and reveal what I honestly don't know—about a headline-grabbing topic can be immensely helpful to an anxious parent. And it's a core part of being a pediatrician. It's part of what I signed up for.

While parents ask hundreds of sticky questions every month—and those questions change as quickly as the nightly news—some questions come up over and over. In this chapter, we'll go through the twenty most common sticky questions that I (like many pediatricians) field every day, and the answers that I give to parents. Happily, as I mentioned, many of these questions do have clear, simple answers.

Ready to play my version of Twenty Questions? Let's hit them, one by one.

1. Should I skip or postpone certain vaccinations for my child until it's absolutely certain that they have no link to neuro-development diseases such as autism? Science has been wrong before.

The answer to this is very simple: no. No, you shouldn't skip or postpone certain vaccinations for fear that vaccines may cause neurodevelopment diseases. Every day, parents ask me if they should be worried about vaccinations, and I unequivocally say yes, they should be worried, but only if their child *misses* a scheduled vaccination. **Vaccinations are critical to good health.** Unfortunately, childhood vaccinations have become a controversial topic among the general public in the last two decades, if not in the medical community. Most of the controversy centers on the unfounded fear that vaccinations (especially the combined measles/mumps/rubella vaccine, or MMR) are linked to autism or other neurodevelopment disorders. **No link has ever been found.**

All the conjecture was caused by one very small published report in the 1990s led by Dr. Andrew Wakefield in London. He announced to the media that he believed the MMR vaccine damaged the intestines, allowing harmful proteins to leak from the gut into the bloodstream and make their way into the brain. Although his paper was published, an association between MMR and autism was *not* proven. Unfortunately, Dr. Wakefield's announcement was enough to cause worldwide panic.

That research has long since been discredited. Since then, ten large scientific studies have found *no evidence* linking vaccinations to autism or any other cognitive disorders. However, the rumors and misinformation simply won't go away.

But during this period, another theory emerged: that autism was caused by thimerosal, a mercury-based preservative used in many vaccines since the 1930s. Again, studies also have found *no link* between thimerosal and autism. However, in this case it hardly matters anymore because in 2001, thimerosal was removed from most childhood vaccines—not because of any link to autism but as a way to decrease children's cumulative exposure to mercury. In fact, since the removal of thimerosal, the number of children with autism has continued to escalate.

Children receive many vaccinations during the first two years of life, and autistic children are often diagnosed during those years, so the two might seem related. But the only connection left between autism and vaccinations is coincidental timing. Just because two things occur at the same time does not mean one caused the other. In the early twentieth century, some people believed that ice cream caused polio. Why? Polio is an enterovirus, a type of virus that is much more likely to cause disease in the summer. And summer is peak ice cream season. So some people wrongly concluded that there was a causal link between polio and eating ice cream.

The bottom line is that childhood vaccinations are safe and critical to good health.

2. Should I "bank" the blood from my newborn's umbilical cord?

If you have a family history of certain diseases, you may be thinking of doing this. The blood from your baby's umbilical cord can be collected just after birth. The stem cells in the cord blood can be separated out, frozen in liquid nitrogen, and used in the future to treat some diseases—such as leukemia, lymphoma, aplastic anemia, severe sickle cell anemia, and severe combined immune deficiency. They can also be used to treat side effects from radiation and chemotherapy, which kill not only cancerous cells but also the good stem cells housed in the bone marrow. The stem cells can be transplanted into the child or another family member, where they produce healthy new blood cells that help boost the immune system and fight the disease.

The only significant risk is to your wallet. A specific kit must be ordered ahead of time from your chosen cord-blood bank at a cost of several hundred dollars. Hospitals charge about $1,000 to $2,000 for collecting the blood from the umbilical cord. Plus there is also a yearly maintenance fee for storing the cord blood. These costs are why the American Academy of Pediatrics (AAP) says banking should be considered only if there is a family member with a current or potential need for a stem cell transplant; otherwise, the AAP worries that cord-blood banks may be preying on the fears of new parents. Another reason not to rush in: Umbilical cord stem cell transplants only work on children or young adults. Full-grown bodies need more blood-forming stem cells than the cord supplies. That's why most bone marrow transplants using cord blood are done on young relatives of a donating child. In fact, there is little experience with transplanting self-donated cells.

Some doctors support saving umbilical cord blood because of the promise stem cell research holds for treating disease—but the truth is, we just don't know if that's going to work out.

My recommendation is (of course!) to talk to your obstetrician or pediatrician about whether this makes sense for you. If it does, ask a lot of questions about the cord-blood banks you're considering. The FDA has set standards for cord-blood collection and storage. You can also donate your child's umbilical cord blood for research or to save the life of another child (though then you can't access it later on). If we all banked our children's cord blood, it would increase the odds of others finding a match. Check out the National Marrow Donor Program for information on donating at www.marrow.org/HELP/Donate_Cord_Blood _Share_Life/index.html.

3. Do I need to clean the umbilical cord stump with alcohol during every diaper change until it falls off?

No, not during *every* diaper change. Just keep the stump *clean* and *dry*.

First-time parents can be hyperconcerned about umbilical cord stumps, probably because these souvenirs of the baby's gestational journey seem alien and a bit bizarre. Shriveled umbilical cords aren't pretty, granted, and many parents are grossed out by them. But checking them during diaper changes for any signs of infection such as redness, oozing, or foul odor is a good habit. Then what should you do?

- Swab it with a cotton ball and alcohol once or twice a day— at most. It's easy to do and may help reduce infection by removing any stubborn crud and killing any germs that migrate from the diaper.
- Of course, do clean around the umbilical cord if it gets soiled from stool, urine, or spit-up.

- Before putting on a fresh diaper, let the cord air-dry.
- Fold the diaper below the umbilical cord or use specifically designed newborn diapers that have a cutout for the umbilical cord.

Many parents also ask me if there's a way to make the umbilical cord fall off faster. Unfortunately the answer is no. It usually drops off in ten to fourteen days no matter what regimen you follow. Of course, in the happy event that the umbilical cord falls off on day nine, there's no harm in thinking that your swabbing routine hastened its exit.

4. Do babies really need to sleep on their backs?

Yes. This is necessary to reduce the risk of sudden infant death syndrome (SIDS). Create this "back to sleep" habit right from the start so your newborn learns that this is the sleeping position.

There is one potential side effect from the child always lying with her head in the same position. The bones in newborns' heads are still forming, so babies can develop flattened heads, a condition called positional plagiocephaly. This is usually only a temporary problem, but some babies may need to wear special head-shaping helmets for a year or undergo physical therapy to correct it.

So, how do you prevent positional plagiocephaly? By turning your baby's head to one side, alternating each night: right facing one night, left facing the next, and so on.

5. Is it better to treat my toddler's ear infection with antibiotics or see if it gets better on its own?

I am so glad parents are asking this question. It tells me that they are aware of the risks of overusing antibiotics. The answer? It depends. If the child is younger than two, has a high fever, is in severe pain, or has underlying chronic medical problems, I usually recommend starting antibiotics.

But about 80 percent of ear infections will heal without an antibiotic. So please don't demand antibiotics. I know it's tempting, especially if your child is miserable and you've taken the morning off from work to visit the doctor. But using antibiotics unnecessarily not only exposes your child to possible side effects from the medication but also encourages antibiotic-resistant bacteria strains, which are becoming a deadlier problem every year in the U.S.

Besides, even kids who are taking an antibiotic for an ear infection will often feel a lot better in twenty-four hours due to the pain medication I've suggested, *not* the antibiotic, which is just starting to work at that point. So if your child is otherwise healthy, try treating the ear infection with pain medication only and schedule a follow-up appointment in two to three days.

However, that follow-up appointment is a *must*, because 20 percent of ear infections will not heal on their own and could lead to a hearing problem or other complications.

6. Can my child really develop a weakened immune system if our house is too clean?

Theoretically, yes. But practically and realistically, no.

This misconception began circulating some years ago, thanks to magazine articles about overzealous parenting (though these probably made people feel better about blowing off housecleaning). If you lived in a sterile environment, your child's immune system would not develop properly. All humans need exposure to common, everyday bacteria, viruses, and garden-variety germs to develop a strong immune system and build up immunities. But unless you clean your house nearly twenty-four hours a day with antibacterial chemicals, rarely let your child outside, shun visitors, and never allow other people to touch your child, you can't stop the necessary germ bombardment.

You can still blow off housecleaning. Just use a different excuse.

7. I found a tick! Should we immediately treat our child for Lyme disease?

It depends on how long the tick has been there.

My family often spends vacations in "high-Lyme" areas (where the ticks that transmit Lyme disease are known to live), so I'm just as worried as many parents are about this bacterial disease, which can cause a rash, fever, joint pain, heart ailments, and nervous system damage (to humans and pets, too). However, some parents are terrified by Lyme disease. Finding a little black bloodsucking hitchhiker on their child's ankle that just might be an *Ixodes dammini* (otherwise known as a deer tick) triggers a panic attack.

Here's some relief: A tick can transmit Lyme disease only if it's been on a human for *at least* twenty-four hours or more. If you are certain that the tick hasn't been on your child that long, you're in the clear. When you're not sure how long the tick has been attached, I may prescribe a course of antibiotics.

Some parents ask if their child should have a Lyme blood test right away. Unfortunately, the common test looks for antibodies to the Lyme bacteria—but they may not show up for several weeks after the tick bite. That's why when no treatment is prescribed, many doctors recommend a blood test about one month after the tick was discovered, just to be sure. Another option is to test the tick. If you saved the tick, it can be sent to a lab to be tested for the Lyme bacteria.

8. Are plastics leaching toxic chemicals into my children's food?

They could be. But the real question is how dangerous the typical daily exposure to these chemicals really is to babies and children—and to us adults, for that matter.

One of the main controversies concerns a chemical called bisphenol A, or BPA, which is used in many plastic bottles, aluminum can linings, and plastic food containers. We've known for years that trace amounts of BPA leach into food and that most people have tiny amounts of BPA in their blood and urine.

We know that BPA can be harmful to living creatures. In animal studies, BPA has been linked to premature puberty, breast and prostate cancer, immune deficiencies, and brain abnormalities. But for years, the evidence in humans has been slim and inconclusive.

Consequently, since the 1980s the Food and Drug Administration has maintained that the typical daily exposure to BPA is probably too low to be dangerous to humans. Many doctors have been skeptical about this, but with all the other clear-cut environmental dangers we deal with daily—secondhand smoke, lead paint, smog, trans fats, mercury, drivers talking on cell phones—BPA didn't seem like the most pressing concern. So it stayed in plastic, and in us.

In 2008, however, BPA started getting more scrutiny and more media attention. Canada banned the use of BPA in all baby bottles, saying that babies, because of their small size, could be at greater risk from even low levels of the chemical. A study in *The Journal of the American Medical Association* found that adults with high levels of BPA in their urine had a high risk of diabetes, heart disease, and liver disease. Then the FDA admitted that the two main studies it had long relied on weren't really solid enough to alleviate fears about the chemical.

We'll be hearing more about BPA. Personally, I try to minimize my family's exposure to plastic food containers in general, and I recommend the same to the parents of my patients. When it comes to a developing fetus, infant, baby, or toddler, reducing exposure to plastics may be especially important, as even minuscule amounts of BPA theoretically could affect their health since their body mass is so low. What I recommend:

Limit the use of plastic food containers for serving or storing food as much as you can. Use glass, paper, and ceramic containers—*especially* for microwaving foods. (See below.)

Never heat a plastic baby bottle in the microwave. And avoid heating food in any plastic container, even if it's marked "microwave safe." Studies have found that heating plastic containers increases the amount of BPA (and other chemicals) that leaches into food.

Memorize "5-4-1-2, all the rest are bad for you." It's a great little mnemonic helper. If you turn plastic bottles and food containers over, you'll usually find numbers on the bottom that indicate the type of plastic they're made from. Plastic containers marked with 5, 4, 1, or 2 contain little or no BPA. Toss anything with any number other than the four digits in the singsongy rhyme above.

Go soft. If you can't locate a number on the bottom of the container, opt for softer, pliable containers. BPA is mostly found in rigid, shatterproof, reusable polycarbonate plastic—the kind used in some CD cases, baby bottles, water bottles, and other hard plastic containers. Softer plastic containers usually contain less of the chemical.

Cut down on cans. Opt for more fresh and frozen foods and fewer canned foods. BPA is used in the plastic lining of many canned foods and beverages, including soup. It's also used in soda cans, which is one more reason to go sparingly on soda. Paper containers for liquids are a better choice.

Use BPA-free pacifiers and baby bottles. More and more of both are on the market.

Relax. When it comes to your baby or toddler, there are more important worries than hard plastics leaching microscopic amounts of chemicals into food. Think about obesity, accidents, swallowing toy parts, and flushing insurance documents down the toilet, for starters. Follow my tips, but don't forget to focus on the big picture.

Skip the Sippy Cup Fad

I constantly see parents handing their children plastic sippy cups of juice to carry around all day. Parents use them as a substitute pacifier. This makes me crazy. Toddlers don't need to sip juice from a cup for five hours while they play, walk, pet the dog, watch TV, and read a book. They don't need the extra calories, the extra tooth decay, or the extra exposure to plastic. You can find sippy cups that are BPA-free, but that's no excuse to keep one attached to your toddler like an appendage. If you choose to give your child a sippy cup to carry around, I suggest filling it with the best sugar-free beverage on earth—water.

9. Should I have my child's lead levels screened?

Yes. I like to start lead screening at eight or nine months of age and do a follow-up every year through kindergarten. The test is a fairly easy finger-stick test that most pediatricians can perform in their office.

Why is yearly lead screening so important? A child's developing brain is extremely susceptible to damage from lead, which can cause problems such as learning disabilities, hyperactivity, shortened attention spans, and even delayed growth or hearing problems. Even very minor lead exposure may have an impact. While the Centers for Disease Control say that lead levels in blood are a concern if they exceed ten ug/dl (ten micrograms per deciliter)—about 2 percent of U.S. children are above this level—we're now finding that even lower levels of lead can cause cognitive trouble. For example, there's mounting evidence linking lead levels under ten ug/dl to subtle drops in IQ. That's worrisome, because about 1.4 million American children have blood lead levels between five and nine ug/dl.

How do children acquire lead poisoning? First, lead is ubiquitous in our environment. It's in our air, water, food, soil, and just about everything you—and your baby—physically encounter. If it's any consolation, you (and your parents) were likely exposed to much greater levels as kids than your own children face today. That's because lead is no longer commonly used in paint and because leaded gasoline—once a huge environmental contributor—has gone the way of the dodo bird. Since automakers switched to unleaded gasoline in the 1970s, the lead levels in children's blood have plummeted. But they haven't dropped to zero. That's because children like to explore, play, and put things in their mouth. These include lead sources such as dirt, paint chips, toys, and other common items that could contain lead. So your goal is to remove as many potential sources of lead from your child's environment as possible. There's no peeling paint in your home or garage? Great. Now do the following:

- **Don't remodel your home if you're pregnant or trying to get pregnant.** Construction kicks up dust that contains lead. The metal could find its way into your system and might affect your unborn baby's development.
- **Do use filtered water for cooking and drinking.** About 20 percent of human exposure to environmental lead comes from municipal water supplies. A good filter on the tap can eliminate 99 percent of the lead in water, not to mention other toxins, including the trace amounts of prescription medications that have been found in municipal water supplies. Boiling water cannot eliminate lead or other toxins.
- **If you can't use a filter, let it flow.** Allow cold water to run from the spigot for two minutes before using it to make baby

formula. (Don't waste the water; fill a few containers and use it for plants, cleaning, etc.)

- **Be wary of soft vinyl lunch boxes.** Remember the good old days when we carried metal lunch boxes? Those days are gone because—wait for it—metal lunch boxes are now considered *dangerous weapons.* Schools banned them, so parents switched to vinyl lunch boxes. But these may be lined with PVC (polyvinyl chloride) and unfortunately, PVC contains lead, which can contaminate food and hands. When this was discovered, some products were recalled. Only buy soft vinyl lunch boxes that have "lead-free" on the packaging. Check out the FDA's website (www.fda.gov) to learn more.
- **Check toys.** The 2008 lead scare from toys made in China caused a sensation. While thousands of tainted toys were pulled from store shelves, no one knows how many remain in the odd toy store here and there, or in day care toy bins, or hidden behind the couch. If you have young children, avoid giving them toys imported from China for the near future, and I especially wouldn't buy any cheap, no-name toys in dollar stores. China has vowed to fix the manufacturing problems that produced lead-contaminated toys, and the U.S. has taken steps to prevent toxic toys from entering the country, so toys should be safer. Still, for updates on toy recalls and other information, check the Consumer Product Safety Commission website at www.cpsc.gov/cpscpub/prerel/category/toy.html.
- **Have a look at the toys in your child's day care center.** If the toys are several years old or falling apart, they could be sources of lead.
- **Avoid candy or gum imported from Mexico.** Many varieties of candy made in Mexico have been found to be tainted with lead. Again, check the FDA's website (www.fda.gov) for more information. Also avoid low-cost bulk candy—the kind often used in pre-made party favors, grab bags, piñatas, and the like—which may be imported and lead contaminated.

- **Limit play on artificial turf.** Wash hands and sneakers well after kids have romped on artificial turf, found in some playgrounds, miniature golf courses, and sports arenas.

Hopefully, your child's lead test will show a lead level lower than three ug/dl. If it's five to ten ug/dl, and you've eliminated all likely sources, talk to your pediatrician about other ways to lower your child's lead exposure. Diet may be a factor; if your child is deficient in iron, calcium, or vitamin C, it can increase lead absorption.

If your doctor sees no other hidden culprits, he or she may just recommend monitoring your child's lead levels more closely to make sure they don't rise. As a parent, your game plan should be to look for potential sources of lead and, whenever possible, eliminate those sources from your child's world as best you can.

10. Should my child eat only organic food?

As you probably know, organic foods are free of pesticides, certain preservatives, and other chemicals commonly used to grow or process food. Eating a largely organic diet can significantly decrease the amount of pesticides and chemicals in our bloodstream. In fact, a study of pregnant women showed that those who ate organic foods reduced the amount of artificial pesticides and chemicals in their blood by 90 percent.

How beneficial is that? We really don't know, but it likely can't hurt. Other research has found that when pregnant women are exposed to large amounts of a common pesticide—organophosphates, used to kill weeds and insects—their babies are at greater risk for having smaller heads, lower birth weights, and developmental abnormalities.

However, research has shown only that *environmental* exposure to organophosphates had these effects. Studies have not yet shown that *ingesting* residual amounts of these chemicals poses a danger to developing fetuses, infants, babies, or adults. Also, no studies to date have proven that eating an organic diet provides any specific health benefits or reduces the risk of any disease.

As more experts in food science continue rigorous, long-term research and studies on organic diets, there may be scientific evidence to prove specific health benefits of eating organic foods sometime in the future. I personally believe that eating an organic diet and decreasing the levels of pesticides in the blood is a good idea—especially if you're even thinking about getting pregnant or already are. Unborn children may be most susceptible to any potential harmful effects of the chemicals in the foods their moms eat. Children under age three, because of their size and their developing brains and nervous systems, are also more likely to be susceptible. So if, budget-wise, it's a question of affording either organic baby food for your toddler or organic peanut butter for your ten-year-old, opt for the former.

And make no mistake, cost is a big issue. Organic food is often twice as expensive as nonorganic, and that can strain family budgets—especially when economic times are less than utopian. Also, no conclusive research has shown that organic foods are more nutritious than their nonorganic counterparts, so if buying organic means that fewer fruits and veggies wind up on your table, then *that is not a good trade-off.* Making sure that your kids receive the minerals, vitamins, and other nutrients they need from fruits and veggies is more important.

Sure, some studies suggest that certain organic foods do indeed pack extra nutrients (in particular, beneficial plant phytochemicals), but I suspect the nutritional differences may be minimal. Your priority is ensuring that your child gets ample helpings of fruits and vegetables every day, organic or not. Fresh is usually best; then I'd strongly opt for frozen over canned. But getting plenty of fruits and vegetables onto your kids' plates—and into their mouths, which can be a bigger challenge—is more important than buying all organic.

Get the Most Organic Bang for Your Buck

If you'd like to incorporate more organic foods into your family's diet, focus on these fruits and vegetables first, as they tend to be the ones that contain the highest levels of pesticides:

* Apples
* Bell peppers
* Berries
* Celery
* Cherries
* Grapes (imported)
* Lettuce
* Nectarines
* Peaches
* Pears
* Potatoes
* Spinach
* Strawberries

11. Is it safe for my child to drink fluoridated water?

Yes.

In recent years, there has been some concern that babies under age one may increase their odds of later developing fluorosis—a relatively harmless condition that can cause faint white lines on tooth enamel—by consuming too much fluoride. This caused some doctors to question whether parents should avoid making baby formula with fluoridated tap water.

Here's what to do: Find out how much fluoride is in your

primary source of drinking water—your pediatrician, dentist, or local water company should be able to tell you this. Based on the levels in the water, you and your doctor will determine a plan of action. Fluorosis is not usually caused just by drinking tap water—it results from the additive effects from multiple fluoride sources. You should always consult with a physician before adding fluoride sources like oral supplements, toothpastes, and mouthwashes.

Though this may all seem a bit tricky to figure out, it's important to remember the benefits of fluoride, such as preventing tooth decay and cavities.

12. My kids love tuna fish. Are they at risk for mercury poisoning?

Only if they are real tuna junkies. High mercury intake from fish can affect a developing nervous system. Avoid white albacore tuna, as it has the highest levels of mercury; opt for canned light tuna instead.

But remember, fish is no enemy! It's a terrific food high in protein and omega-3 fatty acids. Almost all the kids I see need to eat *more* fish, not less. Just monitor the amount you give your children. For young kids, limit fish to twelve ounces per week. Avoid all high-mercury fish, such as swordfish, kingfish, and tilefish, as well as white albacore.

13. Should my child take probiotics?

Foods and supplements that contain live "good" bacteria, called probiotics, have become trendy in the last several years. But what exactly *are* probiotics? They're "live microorganisms, which, when administered in adequate amounts, confer a health benefit on the host," according to the World Health Organization. Foods with added probiotics, such as certain yogurts and other dairy products, are marketed for children (adults, too) in vague terms as "immune system boosters."

There has been a lot of positive research documenting pro-biotic use in children for reducing diarrhea caused by infections or antibiotic use. Probiotics in foods and supplements have been used in Europe for many years for these purposes and are safe. There are many different types of probiotic organisms. There is no one-size-fits-all for all conditions, so it's important not only to use the appropriate probiotic for your child's symptoms but also to use the correct dosage. Talk to your doctor, or check the product's label to make sure you're using the probiotic correctly.

When I recommend probiotics for digestive health, I prefer to prescribe them in supplemental forms (rather than in pre-packaged foods), because the probiotics are much more consis-tent in this form and are generally more effective than probiotics in a food that's been sitting on a shelf or in a refrigerator. This way, too, I know exactly what type of bacteria is being ingested and the amount. BioGaia, which is available as probiotic-coated straws that can be used in any drink, chewables, or drops for in-fants, is one that I prefer for patients. I also recommend Florastor Kids (a tasteless powder that mixes into any beverage) and Cul-turelle (tablets) when appropriate for my patients. Probiotics are available over the counter at most grocery or drug stores.

14. My child has a sore throat. Does she need a strep test?

Maybe. Always call your pediatrician if your child has a sore throat that lasts more than twenty-four hours or is accompanied by fever, headache, rash, stomach pain, or vomiting. Those are the warning signs that you might be dealing with something a little more serious than a garden-variety scratchy throat (which can be relieved with nonmedicated lozenges).

But these symptoms aren't enough to prescribe antibiotics.

Even if I strongly suspect strep, I *always* perform a strep test before prescribing antibiotics. Skipping this step is bad doctoring. Why? The most common cause of sore throats in children is a viral infection, which antibiotics can't treat. So in most cases, antibiotics are useless. The only way to be certain that your child has a strep infection—and genuinely needs antibiotics—is to do a throat culture or a rapid antigen strep test in the office (many pediatricians can do this, but not all).

Many parents are too quick to ask for antibiotics when their child has a sore throat. Using antibiotics unnecessarily . . . by now you've heard it over and over: It's allowing killer bacteria to become resistant to some of our most powerful and most valuable drugs.

Remember that a possible strep infection *must* be evaluated by a doctor because untreated strep throat can cause rheumatic heart disease. While that's rare, truth be known, *that's* really why we prescribe antibiotics for strep throat—to ensure it won't damage the heart.

15. I found a lump in my child's breast! Could my nine-year-old have cancer?

Parents of preteens (children nine to thirteen years old) frequently discover a peanut- or grape-sized lump under one of their children's nipples. It happens most often in girls, but boys experience it too. It feels tender to the child, maybe even painful. Naturally, a worried mom—especially one who's been drilled to do breast self-exams—freaks out and phones her pediatrician. *Is it a tumor?! Is it breast cancer?!*

No. It's likely a breast bud and a natural occurrence in puberty. However, if the lump is extremely painful, growing rapidly, red, secreting a discharge, or accompanied by a fever—or if you're just really freaked out—then you should consult your child's doctor.

16. We're about to take a flight to go on vacation, and my baby is a terrible flier. Should I give her Benadryl (diphenhydramine) so she sleeps?

No! This question is far too common. First, as many people know, regular Benadryl (and other antihistamine formulas containing diphenhydramine) acts like a sedative, and any kind of sedation can be dangerous for young children, especially for children under two. In the worst-case scenario, an accidental overdose of diphenhydramine could cause them to stop breathing.

Second, children under age two are more susceptible to the side effects of diphenhydramine, such as rapid heartbeat, dizziness, headaches, blurred vision, seizures, arrhythmias, and toxic psychosis.

Third, the medication may impart the opposite effect of what you're hoping for. Diphenhydramine is used in many drugstore sleeping pills because sedation and drowsiness are common side effects *in adults.* In children, however, diphenhydramine can act as a stimulant and actually make kids irritable and cranky. Many parents (and nearby air passengers, who are ready to scream themselves) make this unhappy discovery somewhere over the Atlantic.

That pretty much destroys the noble sentiment of "I gave my child Benadryl because I didn't want him to disturb the other passengers."

17. Is it safe to put sunscreen on my one-year-old?

It's generally safe to use sunscreen after babies are six months old. However, keeping babies out of the sun in the first place is a much better idea. When you can't, dressing babies in loose-fitting clothes that offer full coverage (meaning long pants and long-sleeved shirts) and a brimmed hat is the best way to avoid sunburn. If it's too hot for that kind of dressing or you'll be outdoors for an extended period, then sunscreen is necessary.

Avoid a Trip to Hell—and Back

 Flying with a baby? Here are some nonpharmaceutical tips to ease the travel time.

* **Travel at off-peak times.** With luck, the plane will be less crowded.

* **Make sure your child is well rested before boarding the plane . . . or try the reverse!** Take a red-eye flight during your child's normal sleeping time. Some children will sleep all the way through a flight.

* **Bring your child's car seat on the plane.** Its comforting familiarity may be calming.

* **Have plenty of diversions.** DVDs, snacks, crayons, toys, games—whatever you think will staunch a crying fit. If people suggest slipping the little tyke a cough suppressant, allergy medicine, or other drugstore sedative, thank them for the tip and suggest that they get something a little stronger from the flight attendant to blunt their own senses a tad. Nobody likes a screaming baby at forty thousand feet, but when sedatives are concerned, parents need to be more worried about their child's health than about getting dirty looks on a 747.

* **Postpone the trip to next year.** I'm serious. Many parents end up wishing they had. If a journey isn't urgent, delaying it may be the smartest move. Toddlers under two (and sometimes older kids) can be horrible travelers and ruin the excursion. Think hard (and factor in any health issues your baby could have along the way): Is this trip worth it?

Opt for a sunscreen with an SPF of 30 or more that has UVA/UVB protection. I recommend using one that's fragrance-free, hypoallergenic, and uses titanium dioxide or zinc oxide to block the sun's rays. Unlike chemical sunscreens—which are absorbed into the skin and take about thirty minutes to fully work—these mineral-based sunscreens aren't absorbed and start protecting skin immediately. Also, use a sunscreen that does *not* contain an insect repellent (see the next sticky question to learn why). A personal favorite is Blue Lizard Australian Sunscreen for Babies.

Just be sure to test a new sunscreen on a small area of your baby's skin and make sure it doesn't irritate the skin. If you're stuck with nothing but a chemical sunscreen, pretest first and then be sure to apply it *thirty minutes before you go out into the sun.* To avoid irritating your baby's eyes, do not apply sunscreen to the backs of your baby's hands in case he rubs his eyes.

Last, remember to reapply the sunscreen every two hours or so—regardless of what the label says—and especially after any water contact. If you forget this part, a scorching sunburn may result. They're painful and dangerous, and the next few days will be a nightmare.

18. My kids love to play outside, but they get eaten alive by mosquitoes. Is it safe to use bug repellent on them?

Yes, if you're careful with it.

The most effective mosquito repellents contain DEET, which, despite the negative associations with this chemical, is not harmful if used sensibly. More than forty-five years of research and wide use have shown that DEET can be used safely. The rare toxic reactions have been due to excessive exposure. And *not* using an insect repellent in buggy areas can carry its own risks. Repellents lower the odds of contracting insect-borne diseases such as Lyme disease, West Nile, or even malaria in some areas.

Some tips for safe use of insect repellents on babies and children:

- **Never use insect repellent on babies younger than two months old, and only use it when absolutely necessary on children under two years old.** Age matters. If the Costa Rica camping excursion can wait a year, that would be best.
- **Don't use repellents that have DEET concentrations greater than 30 percent on children.** That's too high for young bodies.
- **Use a repellent that's strong enough to do the job for the time needed—no longer.** Specifically, use a repellent that contains the *lowest* concentration of DEET needed to protect your child during the time he or she will be outdoors. For example, a repellent with a 10 percent concentration of DEET will provide protection for about two hours, while one with a 24 percent concentration will provide about five hours of protection.
- **Apply it only once.** Do *not* reapply insect repellent later in the day. DEET is absorbed into your child's skin, and reapplying can increase the odds of toxicity.
- **Don't use products that combine sunscreen and insect repellent.** You need to reapply sunscreen at least every two hours for it to remain effective, but you should not reapply DEET-based insect repellent more than once a day (see above).
- **Apply insect repellent only to exposed skin, avoiding a child's face and hands.** Insect repellent can irritate a child's eyes. And don't bother applying DEET repellents to clothes; it doesn't work on them. (There are other repellents that you can put on clothes.)
- **Don't make your kids bug magnets.** On outdoor days, avoid using scented soaps, lotions, or hair-care products on your child, and don't dress your tyke in brightly colored, flowery clothes—all attract bugs. Also, get kids to play away from flower beds, standing water, or the picnic table; these are places where biting critters like to hang out.

- **Be wary of "natural" insect repellents.** Natural doesn't necessarily mean safer, and few natural products (or home remedies) work for very long. One exception is oil of lemon eucalyptus; some research has found that it repels bugs just as effectively as low concentrations of DEET. However, it is only approved for children over three, and the oil vapor packs a very strong punch, which may be irritating to children.

19. Does my child have to wait thirty minutes after eating before going swimming?

No. This myth has been around since I was a little girl and probably got started centuries before that. The old saw says that a child who has just eaten can get severe stomach or muscle cramps while swimming and drown. It is not impossible, strictly speaking; the process of digestion diverts some blood from the rest of the body, which could theoretically increase the risk of muscle cramping. But there's not a single documented episode of drowning due to swimming on a full stomach in the history of medicine. The American Academy of Pediatrics doesn't recommend any waiting period between eating and swimming. Neither does the American Red Cross. And neither do I.

Now, I don't think I'd want to swim the English Channel after eating Thanksgiving dinner. But I see no reason to stop my

Answer the Phone Poolside, Not Inside

During the summer, always keep a charged cordless phone receiver handy outside if you have a pool. Believe it or not, many children have drowned in the fleeting moments when a parent ran into the house to answer a ringing phone.

youngest child from jumping in the ocean after having a peanut butter sandwich—to the occasional horror of other parents.

I wish we could change the adage from "Wait thirty minutes after eating before swimming" to "Keep two eyes on your children every second they're in the water." That would save many more lives.

20. When is it safe for my child to be discharged from the hospital, and when should I advocate for him to stay or go home?

Seeing your child in a hospital bed with an IV in his arm and a breathing tube in his mouth can be heartbreaking. You likely think, "I'd switch spots with you in a heartbeat, little man, if I could ease your suffering." You likely also think that he would be more comfortable in his own bed, surrounded by all his stuffed animals, and ache to get him home as soon as possible.

Or you could have the reverse reaction: Seeing your child hooked up to a lot of equipment might make you think he needs a *long time* to recuperate in the hospital . . . and you might panic when you hear that he's being released.

Both scenarios are common, and I understand both reactions.

That said, you should trust that your doctor and the medical team caring for your child will keep him in the hospital as long as he *needs to be there,* but they also want to let him go home when he's healthy enough. How long a child is in the hospital depends entirely on his condition and how quickly he responds to treatment. All cases are unique, but generally it's safe for a child to go home if you can answer yes to the following questions:

- Can he eat and drink on his own?
- If he's in any pain, is it mild to moderate and under control?
- If he is taking antibiotics or other meds, can they be taken orally instead of through an IV?
- Does his doctor feel it is safe to go home based on his condition?

- Is his doctor confident he will receive any necessary follow-up care?
- Do you feel comfortable bringing him home?

But you should also be able to answer no to these questions:

- Does he have a fever?
- Is he bleeding?
- Is he struggling to breathe on his own?

If you feel that your child is either being released too soon or being kept in the hospital too long, don't hesitate to tell your pediatrician or the attending physician about your concerns.

CHAPTER 8 POP QUIZ ANSWERS

1. Which statement best describes the evidence about vaccines causing autism? The answer is A—despite relentless rumors, there is no clear cause-and-effect evidence. (Pages 262–63.)

2. Do babies really need to sleep on their backs all the time? The answer is C, yes, *always*—it reduces the risk of SIDS. (Page 266.)

3. When using an insect repellent that contains DEET on a child, which strategy should you follow? The answer is B. In fact, all the other strategies can be dangerous! (Page 283.)

4. Transmission of Lyme disease from a tick may occur . . . The answer is A, only if the wretched thing has been attached to your body for twenty-four hours or more. (Page 268.)

5. When should a child's blood levels of lead be tested? The answer is A. Too many young children remain untested! (Page 271.)

6. If you suspect that your child's persistent sore throat is caused by a strep infection, do you need to go to the pediatrician for a strep culture test?
The answer, again, is A. You *always* need to get a strep culture test before using antibiotics. (Page 279.)

7. What does Dr. Jen personally think of sippy cups? The answer is B. (Page 271.)

Appendixes

Appendix A

Here is a *tiny* sampling of the thousands of actors, athletes, music stars, and other prominent people who have chronic health issues. And to make it more than just another list, I've turned it into a little game: See if you can match up the person with the condition. I've thrown in some easy ones from the annals of history in case your knowledge of sports or pop culture is sketchy. (Hint: When in doubt, choose asthma.)

Conditions

a. Possible Asperger's syndrome (mild form of autism)

b. Asthma

c. Attention deficit/hyperactivity disorder (ADHD)

d. Parent of an autistic child

e. Blind and/or deaf

f. Cancer

g. Diabetes

h. Down syndrome

i. Dyslexia

j. Epilepsy

k. Multiple sclerosis

l. Parkinson's disease or Parkinson's syndrome

m. Spina bifida

n. Stuttering

o. Wheelchair bound

APPENDIX A

Famous People

_____ Muhammad Ali, boxing champion

_____ Christina Applegate, actress

_____ Lance Armstrong, cycling champion

_____ Ludwig van Beethoven, composer and pianist

_____ Halle Berry, actress

_____ Orlando Bloom, actor

_____ Chris Burke, actor

_____ Clive Burr, former drummer for heavy metal band
Iron Maiden

_____ Coolio, rapper and recording artist

_____ Sheryl Crow, recording artist

_____ Tom Cruise, actor

_____ Leonardo da Vinci, artist and scientist

_____ Walt Disney, animator and film producer

_____ DMX, rapper and recording artist

_____ Albert Einstein, scientist

_____ Ernie Els, pro golfer

_____ Mary Jo Fernandez, pro tennis player

_____ Doug Flutie, pro football player

_____ Michael J. Fox, actor

_____ Galileo, scientist

_____ Brenda Gildehaus, champion BMX bike rider

_____ Danny Glover, actor

_____ Tracey Gold, actress

_____ Elvis Grbac, pro football player

_____ Chanda Gunn, Olympic bronze medalist in ice hockey

_____ Stephen Hawking, scientist

APPENDIX A

_____ Salma Hayek, actress

_____ Juwan Howard, pro basketball player

_____ Jim "Catfish" Hunter, pro baseball player and Hall of Famer

_____ James Earl Jones, actor

_____ Helen Keller, author

_____ Jason Kidd, pro basketball player

_____ Keira Knightley, actress

_____ Ricki Lake, talk show host

_____ Lindsay Lohan, actress

_____ Greg Louganis, Olympic gold medalist in diving

_____ Marlee Matlin, actress

_____ John Cougar Mellencamp, recording artist

_____ Rodney Peete, pro football player

_____ Michael Phelps, Olympic swimming champion

_____ Pink, recording artist

_____ Keanu Reeves, actor

_____ Julia Roberts, actress

_____ Franklin Delano Roosevelt, thirty-second U.S. president

_____ Emmitt Smith, pro football player

_____ Alison Streeter, English Channel swimmer (more than forty crossings)

_____ Harriet Tubman, abolitionist

_____ Dominique Wilkins, pro basketball player

_____ Montel Williams, talk show host

_____ Stevie Wonder, recording artist

_____ Kristi Yamaguchi, Olympic gold medalist in figure skating

_____ Neil Young, recording artist

ANSWERS

Possible Asperger's syndrome (mild form of autism)

Albert Einstein, scientist

Asthma

DMX, rapper and recording artist
Coolio, rapper and recording artist
Mary Jo Fernandez, pro tennis player
Juwan Howard, pro basketball player
Jim "Catfish" Hunter, pro baseball player and Hall of Famer
Ricki Lake, talk show host
Lindsay Lohan, actress
Greg Louganis, Olympic gold medalist in diving
Pink, recording artist
Emmitt Smith, pro football player
Alison Streeter, English Channel swimmer (more than forty crossings)
Dominique Wilkins, pro basketball player
Kristi Yamaguchi, Olympic gold medalist in figure skating

Attention deficit/hyperactivity disorder (ADHD)

Jason Kidd, pro basketball player
Michael Phelps, Olympic gold medalist in swimming
Tracey Gold, actress

Possible but unconfirmed ADHD

Leonardo da Vinci, artist and scientist
Walt Disney, animator and film producer
Galileo, scientist

Parent of an autistic child

Ernie Els, pro golfer
Doug Flutie, pro football player
Rodney Peete, pro football player

Blind and/or deaf
Ludwig van Beethoven, composer and pianist
Helen Keller, author
Marlee Matlin, actress
Stevie Wonder, recording artist

Cancer
Christina Applegate, actress (breast cancer)
Lance Armstrong, cycling champion (testicular cancer)
Sheryl Crow, recording artist (breast cancer)

Diabetes
Halle Berry, actress

Down syndrome
Chris Burke, actor

Dyslexia
Orlando Bloom, actor
Tom Cruise, actor
Salma Hayek, actress
Keira Knightley, actress
Keanu Reeves, actor

Epilepsy
Chanda Gunn, Olympic bronze medalist in ice hockey
Danny Glover, actor
Harriet Tubman, abolitionist
Neil Young, recording artist

Multiple sclerosis
Clive Burr, drummer for heavy metal band Iron Maiden
Brenda Gildehaus, champion BMX bike rider
Montel Williams, talk show host

Parkinson's disease or Parkinson's syndrome
Muhammad Ali, boxing champion
Michael J. Fox, actor

Spina bifida
Elvis Grbac, pro football player
John Cougar Mellencamp, recording artist

Stuttering
James Earl Jones, actor
Julia Roberts, actor

Wheelchair bound
Stephen Hawking, scientist (due to amyotrophic lateral sclerosis, or
    ALS, also known as Lou Gehrig's disease)
Franklin Delano Roosevelt, thirty-second U.S. president (due to polio)

Appendix B

The Five Disorders That Make Up the Autism Spectrum

1. **Autistic disorder (or autism)** is the most common disorder found on the autism spectrum. Impairments range from mild to severe and affect social interaction, communication, behavior, interests, and activities, and may also involve developmental delays.

2. **Asperger's syndrome** is sometimes referred to as "mild autism," meaning it's on the higher-functioning end of the spectrum. Still, impairments and symptoms may range from mild to severe. Children with Asperger's syndrome primarily have trouble with social and communication skills, but their intelligence levels are generally average to superior. As adults, many have satisfying careers and successful relationships; some have written books about their disorder. It's often rumored that Albert Einstein had Asperger's, and there are compelling arguments for this, but diagnosing long-gone figures is notoriously difficult. There's simply too much guesswork involved.

3. **Pervasive developmental disorder–not otherwise specified (PDD-NOS)** has been described as "kind of like autism, but not meeting enough criteria to qualify for the autism diagnosis," by multiple sources. Okay, so what does that mean? It means that people with PDD-NOS display autistic-like symptoms (generally problems with communication and/or being intensely preoccupied with certain activities), but there may not be many symptoms or any severe ones.

4. **Childhood disintegrative disorder (CDD):** Children with CDD develop normally until they're three or four (sometimes older) but then dramatically regress, losing language, social, and self-help skills, including loss of

bowel and bladder control, and may also develop seizures. Eventually, the child may display autistic characteristics, including mental retardation. CDD is very rare and the least common form of ASD.

5. **Rett syndrome** is known to be genetic and primarily affects girls. Children with Rett generally have impaired speech, language, and motor skills, particularly with the hands and, in some cases, with walking and balance. They may also have mild to severe learning disabilities.

Acknowledgments

Jennifer Trachtenberg, MD

From the bottom of my heart I would like to thank all who have helped make this book a reality. It goes without saying; I could not have done it alone.

First, I'd like to thank Joint Commission Resources and The Joint Commission, who approached me to collaborate on this project. I am still in awe that they chose me to partner with them. I would specifically like to thank Victoria Gaudette for her editorial savvy and endless hours working with me on the book and for trusting and valuing my medical opinions. A big thank-you also goes to Cathy Hinckley for her confidence in me as a pediatrician and author. For their tremendous support in developing this book, I'd also like to thank Karen Timmons, CEO of Joint Commission Resources, and Mark Chassin, M.D., CEO of The Joint Commission.

Thank you to my team (and friends) at RealAge who always support me and my endeavors 100 percent. A big thanks to Andy Mikulak, Meredith Wade, Carol Valdez, and my agent, Candice Fuhrman. I must give an extra special thank-you to Val Weaver—a tremendous editor and friend—who has the ability to take my thoughts and transform them so eloquently into words. I couldn't do any of this without her finesse. I'd also like to thank Drs. Mehmet Oz and Mike Roizen for paving the path for this book by coauthoring *You: The Smart Patient* with The Joint Commission.

I am also grateful to Eileen Norris and Ron Geraci for writing this book with me. Their contributions allowed me to focus on the medical content while they worried about the organizational details and extra elements you'll find throughout the book.

I'd like to thank the publishing team at Free Press, especially my editor, Dominick Anfuso, and his assistant Leah Miller, who guided me through this endeavor and believed in the importance and relevance of this book for parents.

Thanks, also, to my colleagues at Carnegie Hill Pediatrics—Stephanie Freilich, MD; Neal Kotin, MD; Harold Raucher, MD; Barry Stein, MD; and Melissa Goldstein, MD—for their camaraderie and medical expertise, which has enabled me to continually learn from them and better myself as a pediatrician.

A special thanks goes out to my patients and their parents, who allow me to care for them and believe in my abilities as a pediatrician and a mom. Hopefully, I have taught them the importance of a "medical home" where no questions are silly and where medical knowledge is empowering and not something to fear. My hope is that this book will help parents whom I am not able to see in my practice.

Last, but certainly not least, hugs and kisses to my family, especially my husband David and my three wonderful children, Noah, Eric, and Emily. Though I knew since I was just a child myself that I wanted to be a doctor and spend my time caring for and helping others, nothing at all compares to my satisfaction of being your mommy. Love you lots.

The Joint Commission and Joint Commission Resources

This guide is dedicated to leaders, physicians, nurses, pharmacists, and other staff at health care organizations in the United States who work daily to heal the sick and injured and who are passionately committed to patient safety and quality care. In particular, we recognize those who strive to provide the best care and treatment for children, who are indeed our future and our country's greatest asset.

We would also like to acknowledge the staff of The Joint Commission and Joint Commission Resources, whose work contributes to the welfare of patients by supporting health care organizations in their quality and safety efforts.

Finally, special thanks to our partners in this book, Dr. Jennifer Trachtenberg and RealAge, for their efforts and dedication to improving health care. And thanks to our colleagues at Free Press for helping us to share these important messages about patient safety and quality health care with the public.

Mark Chassin, M.D.
President
The Joint Commission

Karen H. Timmons
President
Joint Commission
Resources

Index

About the Authors

Jennifer Trachtenberg, MD, author of *Good Kids, Bad Habits: The RealAge Guide to Raising Healthy Children*, serves as chief pediatric officer for RealAge.com. A nationally renowned parenting expert and board-certified pediatrician, she has practiced pediatric and adolescent medicine for more than sixteen years and maintains a successful private pediatric practice in New York City. She is also assistant clinical professor in pediatrics at The Mount Sinai Medical Center, a fellow of the American Academy of Pediatrics, and the mother of three children. Dr. Jen has appeared on NBC's *Today* show and CNN's *Headline News*, among other programs. She has written articles on various health and parenting topics, including child development and childhood obesity.

For almost sixty years, **The Joint Commission,** a private, not-for-profit organization, has been the nation's leader in continuously improving patient safety and health care quality. The Joint Commission is the principal standards setter and evaluator for a variety of health care organizations, including hospitals, ambulatory care, behavioral health care, home care, laboratories, and long-term care. Joint Commission accreditation is the coveted Gold Seal of Approval™ and means that a health care organization complies with the most rigorous standards of performance. And that means safe and quality health care for *you.*

Joint Commission Resources (JCR) is the publishing, educational, and consulting not-for-profit affiliate of The Joint Commission. JCR provides practical, solutions-oriented information on health care quality, medical error prevention, infection prevention and control, medication management, and facility safety to health care organizations around the world. The World Health Organization designated The Joint Commission and Joint Commission International (a division of JCR) as a Collaborating Centre on Patient Safety Solutions to identify, develop, and disseminate strategies which will reduce or eliminate the occurrence of errors in health care organizations.

This book, *The Smart Parent's Guide to Getting Your Kids Through Checkups, Illnesses, and Accidents,* represents The Joint Commission's and JCR's second book specifically for the public. The first book, *YOU: The Smart Patient,* coauthored with Drs. Michael F. Roizen and Mehmet C. Oz and also published by Free Press, was a *New York Times* best seller and a Quill Book Award nominee. It was featured on the *Today Show* and *Oprah* and in *Redbook, Real Simple, Good Housekeeping,* and *Reader's Digest,* among other popular media.

Visit us on the Web at www.jointcommission.org and www.jcrinc.com.

RealAge.com is a healthy-lifestyle website that inspires its members to "Live Life to the Youngest" and to pursue their health and wellness goals by making their RealAge younger. The site offers the patented RealAge Test, the most widely used method for measuring overall health, and is an online home of the YOU Docs, Michael Roizen, MD, and Mehmet Oz, MD, and their bestselling RealAge and YOU books. Over 30 million people have measured their RealAge by taking the RealAge Test and have received a personalized plan to make their RealAge younger. This leading healthy-lifestyle website also features more than 65 additional health-risk assessments, as well as health tips and information, all backed by current medical science. RealAge.com is a wholly owned subsidiary of Hearst Magazines, a division of the Hearst Corporation.

Eileen Norris has been a Chicago-area journalist for more than twenty-five years. She has been a contributing writer and/ or editor for four health books, the latest as ghostwriter for a doctor-authored book on parenting. She helped to develop and manage *YOU: The Smart Patient* by Drs. Mehmet Oz and Mike Roizen and The Joint Commission (Free Press, 2006). She served as a writer for *The Harvard Medical School Family Health Guide* (Simon & Schuster, 1999), and as managing editor for *The American Medical Association's Complete Medical Encyclopedia* (Random House, 2003). As a specialist in health and medical issues, her work has been featured in *Prevention,* the Harvard Health Letter, and *Arthritis Today,* as well as general interest publications such as *Newsweek* and the *Chicago Tribune.* A former editorial manager in publications at Joint Commission Resources, she began her career as a reporter for the *Chicago Tribune.*

Ron Geraci is a well-known writer who worked extensively on Drs. Mehmet Oz and Michael Roizen's bestselling book *YOU: The Smart Patient.* He covered the gamut of health topics as a former editor and columnist at *Men's Health* magazine, and as an editor for *AARP The Magazine.* His popular column "This Dating Life" appeared in *Men's Health* magazine for three years. Geraci's memoir, *The Bachelor Chronicles,* was published in 2006. Geraci served as the editorial consultant for the Discovery Health show *Strictly Dr. Drew.* He also helped lead the creation of a men's channel for Weight Watchers.com, which launched in March 2007. He has appeared on the *Today Show,* CBS's *Early Show, CBS Evening News, Weekend Today,* MSNBC's *Morning Joe,* CNN Health, and several other television programs. Geraci has written for numerous magazines including *Cosmopolitan, Details, Fitness, GQ, Glamour, Marie Claire, Men's Health, Reader's Digest, Redbook, Seventeen, Shape,* and others.

Printed in the United States
By Bookmasters